Your body wants to be healthy!

Every human being has a built-in "blueprint" for good health—for vitality and well-being, for resistance to disease of all kinds.

But most of us spend our lives tearing up this blueprint—with deadly living and eating patterns!

With a wealth of informative and fascinating detail drawn from forty years of clinical observation, testing and treatment at the famed Page Clinic in St. Petersburg Beach, Florida, Dr. Melvin E. Page and his collaborator reveal his basic program for capturing good health—report on dramatic cases of recovery from advanced stages of disease—show how heredity and diet combine to determine your health—and make it undeniably clear that

YOUR BODY IS YOUR BEST DOCTOR!

YOUR BODY IS YOUR BEST DOCTOR!

Melvin E. Page, D.D.S. and H. Leon Abrams, Jr.

Keats Publishing Inc.   New Canaan, Connecticut

YOUR BODY IS YOUR BEST DOCTOR

Third printing, May, 1976

Printed in the United States of America

ISBN Number: 87983-021-2

Pivot Health Books are published by Keats Publishing, Inc.
212 Elm Street, New Canaan, Connecticut 06840

Remember that no doctor ever cured anything. If a patient is cured it is because his own body does it. The doctor helps by his knowledge and aid.

If the efficiency of a person's chemistry is zero, then he is dead. If it is 100 per cent, he is very much alive. Most of us vary between 40 per cent and 70 per cent of the efficiency we should have.

What we in this country are going through has happened before. Toynbee states that in the last 10,000 years there have been 34 civilizations of which only four are in existence today. And these are on the way out.

One thing all of these civilizations had in common shortly before they vanished; they became prosperous. Their material progress overwhelmed them. Maybe this civilization will not go the way of the others if enough of us learn the "why" of degeneration and the "how" of regeneration.

Remember surgery removes a result but does not change the cause.

Civilization, ours as well as probably all others in the past, has been a development of technology by the few, and an education of the many in its use. The result is disasterous to man, because his intelligence has not increased correspondingly. Since we can't increase intelligence except by selective breeding, we must enlarge the field of education to make us aware of the dangers of civilization. Not more education in the uses, but the abuses of technology.

M. E. P.

Contents

Introduction: Health vs. Disease

The morning was bright and fresh as John Dowers left for the golf course to go through 18 holes. Mr. Dowers didn't feel too spry, but otherwise he thought that he was "sitting on top of the world." Yes, he was successful, owned a fine new home, was an executive in a large corporation, had money in the bank and a fine wife and three children. "What more could a man want," he thought to himself. "Yes, life is wonderful," he said as he entered the Country Club golf course. After about twenty minutes on the golf course he felt a sudden, sharp pain in his chest and slumped to the ground. His friends rushed to him but he was pronounced dead upon the arrival of an ambulance. Yes, a coronary at the age of 48, and John Dowers was dead, done for. His friends shook their heads and said that poor old John had been working too hard, driving himself too much—the cause of his coronary was due to stress and strain. But was it? Are coronaries and such degenerative diseases due to stress and strain caused by the so-called tensions of the modern world? The answer is emphatically no, but the cause is still due to the modern world in which John lived.

He had his teeth filled and except for a fleeting thought, never dwelled on the question of what caused his teeth to decay. Then, only eight years earlier, he lost his teeth due to abscesses of the roots. He was just one of the unlucky ones, so he told himself. And then there was the problem of excessive weight which became particularly noticeable in his late thirties; it bothered him a little but he passed it off with the statement that it's just "the middle age spread." What should have puzzled him was the fact that he was not a big eater and if anything, was eating less than when he was younger. Anyway, he thought, the important thing in life was to get ahead and one had to accept slowing up as one got older. He had read the statistics that gave the average man in the U. S. a life span of some 60 years, so what did he have to worry about—there were many more productive and fruitful years ahead and he had a family to raise and educate. But now, John Dowers was dead; his family was left all alone. It would be harder for them now that the bread winner was gone. Sure there was insurance and a few securities, but not enough to provide as dear old dad had. Mary, his wife, now blamed herself for not insisting that John slow up and take things more easily.

Such was only wishful thinking because John had been abusing his body for so long that rest, though desirable, probably wouldn't have made much difference.

John had his warning years ago with the first dental decay, but unfortunately he didn't know that. And, how could he? No one had ever told him and he had never read anything about the subject as little or nothing had been written on the subject. He was largely a victim of the times, but now, fortunately, the picture is beginning to change. One can know if he is willing to search and do some thinking. It is true, as most all dentists know, that tooth decay is an indication of more serious degenerative trouble to come.

This fact may seem strange at first, but when it is realized that the mouth is merely a part of the whole body, that the same blood goes to it that goes to all other parts of the body, and that it consists of cells, living tissue and bone just as the rest of the body, the conclusion becomes fairly obvious.

The tragedy of John's case is that it was avoidable, being a typical degenerative disease. Men of science have been very successful in combating, controlling and immunizing against diseases caused by germs, but they have not as yet done much to alleviate the ravages of degenerative diseases.

Let us look at the case of a certain farmer and his herd of cattle which he had just inherited from an uncle. He was very happy over this good luck because he felt that all of his problems were solved; yes sir, he was sitting on top of the world. He and his family could now feel assured of a nice income from the sale of prime beef cattle. But his glee was short lived. He found that eighteen per cent of the female cattle of the herd could not produce calves and of those that could more than fifty per cent could not nurse their calves. He further found that many of his bulls were impotent. A large proportion of his herd were subjected to fits, and fifty per cent of the bulls died in the prime of life from heart attacks and circulatory conditions. Thirty per cent of the herd was so crippled with arthritis and rheumatism that they could move about only with pain and risk. Further examination revealed that seventy-five per cent of them had teeth that were loose in their jaws, while ninety-five per cent had rotten and missing teeth which caused much difficulty in chewing food. Twenty per cent of the herd was afflicted and dying with cancer.

Obviously the farmer had inherited a liability but he could at least dispose of the cattle. The irony of the above parable is that the figures just quoted belong to the population of the United States. They are the percentages of a number of the most prevalent degenerative diseases that cripple, kill and afflict the people of our country. It is not hard to realize this when you stop and go over the list of people you know who are suffering with such diseases or who have died from them.

In 1958 each man, woman and child in the United States spent an average of $95.00 on medical care which represents the staggering total of 16.7 billion dollars. One of the sad facts concerning this stupendous amount of money for medical care is that it went largely for cure, not for prevention. And many of the ills could have been prevented. Even a healthy body, when it is kept healthy, is

not susceptible to diseases caused by germs as is an unhealthy body. We all know that we have been exposed to
tuberculosis but that most of us didn't develop it. It seems
to attack and get a hold on those bodies that are not in a
good condition of health. The healthy body has resistance
and can fight off the disease, but an unhealthy body rapidly gives in to the attackers and becomes sick. Actually,
many people have sick bodies without realizing it; that is
why they catch colds so easily, or are so susceptible to a
whole host of infectious diseases. As one doctor has stated, "there is never a sick man until he gets down on his
back."

People do not think about their health until they are
sick. Then they run to a doctor and hope for a cure. Prevention is a comparatively new field and until recently
consisted only in immunization. Now, there are campaigns
against cigarettes—the cause of lung cancer—against obesity—found in diabetics—high blood pressure, heart disease, etc. These are a start in the right direction. Premature degenerative diseases can be prevented, in some cases
stopped or even reversed.

We like to think of our bodies as things in which we live
temporarily, things which are really chemical laboratories
and also mechanical miracles. When these bodies function
properly we have excellent health and they are wonderful
places in which to live, but when their functions are impaired and they thus become unhealthy, they can be like
burdens and prisons and cause a great deal of suffering.

It behooves us to take proper care of these dwelling
places so that we can get the greatest possible efficiency
from them and at the same time enjoy them as pleasurable
dwelling places. It is necessary for us to realize their value
to us and to provide the proper care and food so that their
value does not decrease. To do this, it is important to select those foods that supply all the things that are needed
to maintain a healthy body, and also to leave out those
foods and beverages which are harmful. This is admittedly
somewhat difficult because we live in a world of people

who habitually break these rules of good diet because they know nothing of them.

This problem of health is pretty much the same as the one in the Biblical parable of the three brothers each of whom was given twenty talents of silver. One brother squandered his, another buried his, and only the third one used his wisely so that it might increase and make him a better man. So it is with health; we should not squander it, but many do. We should not coddle it, but quite a few people do to little or no avail, for in order to hold on to good health and maintain it the body must be used and nourished wisely so as to provide and increase the good life of joy and happiness.

Primitive man depended upon his instincts of taste, smell and thirst to control his food intake. Nature might have been stingy in her supply at times, but at least the food was wholesome and health building. Primitive man's life was not endangered by what he ate because he ate natural foods. Health was his if violence was avoided. Today the case is almost reversed. Man has learned how to cope with the elements for the most part and with the germ-causing diseases, but with degenerative disease, which is on the rapid increase, man is on the losing side.

The lack of this control is proving to be man's undoing in many fields. Yet the solution to this problem is readily available and only waiting for man to take hold of it and apply it. Why not tackle this problem of health with the same intelligence which we use to regulate forces outside ourselves? It is time we brought intelligence to bear in consideration of the matters of food intake and utilization.

We should not only consider what we eat but also its quality. Does it have the needed ingredients for sustaining optimum nutrition? One should further realize that if the body lacks those necessary things, the end result will be poor health.

Surely man having exercised his mind on the problems of high acreage production, artificial coloring of foods, processing of foods, packaging of foods, and transportation of foods, should now turn some of his attention to the building qualities of food. Some alterations in present food production will have to be made and some temporary economic maladjustments will be felt, but such things have happened before in great periods of industrialization and technological advancement. It is only by such advances and adjustments that man's standard of material existence has been raised to its present high level.

Let's tackle the fundamentals of civilized man's problems. The breakdowns within our bodies lie within our own control provided we achieve an understanding of the physiological processes and needs of our bodies, and provided that we pay the price of self-discipline to meet these fundamental needs.

In some forty years of interest, research, and clinical dental practice with the problem of degenerative disease, I have found that nutrition is the controlling factor. This new concept of dental medicine avails itself of the modern techniques of medicine and the other related sciences.

Good health and cures are often brought about merely by correcting body chemistry. In this approach, the patient must be treated not just for the specific part of the body which noticeably ails him, but for his entire body since each minute part is merely an interacting part of the whole. When body chemistry is functioning properly, one has good health—hence resistance to disease is at its maximum with the result that the body is more able to effectively resist and fight illness.

I. Your Blueprint of Construction

Each individual is a person unto himself and no two individuals are identical. Our biological characteristics, our physical characteristics, were determined by our heredity. When we say heredity, we speak of that inheritance that has made each individual, the uniting of two sex cells, an egg from the female, a sperm from the male. Had it been the same egg and a different sperm, the person would be different entirely. The miracle of all this is that of millions, one particular egg and one particular sperm unite to form one particular person. Of course, heredity is not destiny though many people write and speak of heredity as if it were. For example, each individual is endowed by heredity with a potential height, but this does not mean that he will attain that height or possibly surpass it. Environment plays a vital part. Due to starvation or malnutrition, the individual may be stunted. Likewise, due to malfunction of the glandular system, further stimulated by diet, he may grow to be taller than was his endowed heredity. Both conditions in this respect are abnormal and unhealthful. It is a well known fact, stated and verified by leading scientists, dental and medical authorities, that nutrition, health conditions and exercise are all part of the environment and greatly influence the growth and physical development of children. This in turn, quite naturally, influences the personality development of children. The question is somewhat irrelevant, but it still keeps coming up: Which is more important, heredity or environment? The stock answer to that question is to ask this question: Which is more important, your heart or your lungs? One without the other of course is worthless. The same is true with respect to heredity. Heredity and environment go hand in hand, and we are products of the interaction of the two. Seldom, perhaps never, is either perfect. But when both are within the so-called normal range, that person should grow up as a normal child and mature to normal adulthood.

Often, one deficiency can compensate for another. This is one of the main phases of study of the healing arts. Unfortunately, little is known about those hereditary tendencies that make one person prone to certain degenerative processes while another person may have a stronger constitution and not be so susceptible. The answer is in the heredity of the individual. Still, a person with a wonderful physical heredity can destroy this constitution by bodily abuse such as constantly feeding on a deficient or harmful diet.

But it is now time to turn to the degenerative diseases which are taking so many lives each year. The answer lies primarily within the endocrine structure of the individual which is hereditary, though the endocrine system of a person may be modified, corrected, adjusted, or changed for better or worse, depending upon how one has treated his body since birth.

We are all familiar with diabetes which only a few decades ago was usually fatal. Today it is a serious disease but not at all fatal, nor does it prevent one who is so afflicted from leading a normal life. These people can not retain or even utilize the sugars that they eat in their food, so the sugars are passed from the body in the urine. A certain amount of blood sugar is necessary to sustain life. Therefore diabetics are in danger of a coma and even death. In 1920 insulin was discovered. This hormone was found to be the answer for most diabetics. The disease has other contributing causes, but a malfunctioning pancreas is the most common.

A normal body makes its own insulin, but the heredity of a person with diabetes has given him a pancreas that is incapable of producing sufficient insulin. When insulin is administered by injection, diabetes may be controlled. When you meet a person so afflicted you probably will not suspect, unless you are told by the person concerned, that he has a diabetic heredity because he has created for himself an artificial environment by taking his insulin from outside his own body. Diabetes is the most dramatic and widely known of the disorders of the endocrine glands. Most of us are born with some glands not 100 per cent perfect, yet they are good enough to get us through life, in most cases very well.

All degenerative diseases are a result of malfunctioning of the endocrine and exocrine glands, either due to heredity or damage by environment, (primarily due to a bad diet, or a combination of the two factors which is more common).

The science of genetics, which concerns itself with the study of heredity and just how it works, is rather young. The initial discovery, which is one of the most dramatic stories in the whole history of science, took place in a rather unexpected place, not in a university or a great scientific laboratory, but in a monastery garden in Czechoslovakia between the years of 1857 and 1865. During those years a Roman Catholic monk, Gregor Mendel, worked and experimented methodically in crossing various varieties of the garden pea, carefully noting and studying the differences through several generations. In 1865 Mendel delivered a learned paper on his experiments and findings to the Society of Naturalists in the town of Brno, and the following year this was published in the journal of the Society. Of all the outstanding discoveries of modern science, Mendel's is one of the greatest, although scientists of his time paid no attention to his findings. Mendel was made abbot of the monastery and with his increased responsibilities, he did not pursue his discoveries further. He did not need to; he had made the first great initial discovery of the laws of heredity. His was the key to all further discoveries. It was as if he had opened the eyes so that sight was there, yet everyone refused to look and see. Toward the latter part of the 19th century, scientists began an earnest search into the mysteries of the workings of the laws of heredity. In 1900, sixteen years after the death of Mendel, three European scientists, working independently and not aware of the other's research, made the same discovery that Mendel had made years earlier. At that time Mendel's publication was dug out from the stacks of the library and dusted off, and at last he was posthumously honored and it was decided that this great discovery would henceforth be known as the "Mendelian Laws of Heredity."

The fundamental laws, or rules, of heredity discovered by Mendel are universal in their application to all living things. The significant essence of Mendel's discovery is in his identification of the units of heredity which are called genes and are found in the chromosomes. Each human sex cell is made up of 24 chromosomes which in turn contain thousands of genes, the exact number not being known. It is these genes which give us our traits, brown or blue eyes, brown or blond hair, and so on. The possible combinations of the chromosomes of the sperm, from the male, and of the egg, from the female, run into the millions. With these many possibilities, it is amazing that brothers and sisters are as much alike as they are in many cases, yet we all know of brothers and sisters who are not very much alike. The only people who have identical heredity are identical twins, who come from the same egg and sperm, yet because of environment, they are not exactly identical even though their heredity is the same. To get some idea of heredity, the following simple and classical example is given. Suppose that we cross a white Andulusian chicken with a black one. The offsprings of this mating will all be blue. Then in the third generation, the blue offsprings are crossbred, their offsprings will be as follows: one-fourth will be white, one-fourth will be black, and one-half will be blue. The result is the basic Mendelian ratio of one to one, in the offsprings. Now, in humans, the workings of genetic combinations of genes is very complicated but it still follows, in essence, this basic pattern. With chickens one characteristic is dealt with above, namely color. Now, every living animal is made up of multiple characteristics, so it is easy to see that whereas individuals having the same parents may have many characteristics in common, others will be different, and many of these are not even noticeable on the surface. It is from our parents directly, and from them indirectly, that we get all of our characteristics from our ancestors. If our ancestors carry genes for weak glands, then weakness will be passed on to at least some of the descendants depending upon the alignment of hereditary carriers, genes. That is why one child in a family may be born perfectly healthy while another is not. This then brings us back to endocrinology and the problem of susceptibility to degenerative diseases. Due to heredity, many people are born with malfunctioning glands and they are thus destined to have bad health unless the situation is remedied. One of the most obvious examples of this is the diabetic; this glandular defect is due to the lack of functioning of the isles of Langerhans of the pancreas. With the other glands, the malfunction may not be so readily obvious.

It is the purpose of the blueprint of construction, technically termed the Page anthropometric hypothesis, which has been worked out over a period of years with some 40,000 measurements to indicate the hereditary glandular condition with which an individual was born. The same thing can be accomplished by blood analyses alone, but entails about fifty to sixty blood analyses over a period of a year or more. This is expensive and time consuming for both patient and physician. When the results of the measurements along with blood analyses are utilized, rapid diagnosis is possible and usually response to treatment is quick, depending upon the specific circumstances of each given patient. In this manner, it is usually possible to work out a program that will bring about balanced body chemistry.

Since cavities were thus shown to be related to the systemic conditions of a given individual, it seemed logical that the degree of dental decay would be in direct proportion to the degree of variance from the normal of body metabolism. But the usual method of measuring body metabolism (by measurements of oxygen intake) seemed too inaccurate for this purpose, It is affected by too many external factors. However, as the endocrines control growth through assimilation, their dysfunction should register in bodily proportions. In studying the types of endocrine dysfunction certain rules as to placement of weight were discovered to apply to each. One group was found to have greater weight above the waist while the opposite group had it below the waist. By finding the relative proportion between the upper and lower body measurements it was possible to determine the extent of endocrine dysfunction.

This whole process is one of chemistry in which the glands operate as the thermostats, catalysts, and regulators of bodily functions. By plotting these figures on a chart, along with the amount of dental caries in each case it was found that the degree of bodily disproportion was in direct proportion to dental decay. The forearm was measured from the wrist joint to the elbow and this figure divided by four. Beginning at the wrist and at equally spaced intervals, five circumferential measurements were taken with a narrow cloth tape. This resulted in a wrist measurement, an elbow measurement, and three measurements between. Care was taken to bend the forearm at about 45 degrees to the upper arm so that the point of the elbow would be prominent.

The leg was measured in like manner from the ankle bone to the knee cap, having the knee flexed at the same angle as the elbow, and five measurements at equal intervals were taken. Each leg measurement was divided by the corresponding arm measurement and the result tabulated in a column. These five quotients were added and the result divided by five. This gave a figure which in most cases lay between 1.300 and 1.700 for females.

Measurements taken of these people who had perfect

metabolism during and after the growing age showed about the same results. The figure was about 1.420 for the female. Measurements for the male with perfect metabolism are somewhat less or at about 1.345.

Measurements resulting in a figure less than 1.420 for the female indicates that her metabolism is abnormal with respect to the break down glands, while figures more than 1.420 indicate abnormality with regard to the build up glands. Most all measurements fall between 1.000 and 1.700 for both men and women. The average starting point for the female is 1.550 and for the male it is 1.475, however, a normal graph may start at any point for a specific individual.

These measurements, having been refined over the years from some 40,000 measurements, are then plotted upon the graph-chart especially designed for this particular purpose. The graph then indicates the type of glandular structure with which the individual was born. One abnormal gland upsets the whole structure and thus affects the total metabolism of the body to some degree. Correction of this abnormality then brings about normal functioning body metabolism. Through this method, each person will then have his own particular blueprint of construction, and if glandular supplement is indicated, it is for that person alone and no one else. That is why in this approach to good health, termed body chemistry, each individual is treated as a person and not as a number or statistic. The glandular supplement for a given patient must be determined through very exact blood analysis, urine analysis and other scientific techniques of the healing arts.

All this helps to classify the patient and serves to indicate to a degree the type of diseases to which this patient has been or is susceptible. Diagnosis cannot be made by measurement alone, for metabolism can change over a period of years. A patient in the forties may present measurements of one type and yet be of another dominant type. In a young person, in the teens or twenties, the measurements are almost always trustworthy as an indication of the present metabolism. Most changes from one type of metabolism to the other take place at puberty and menopause, or as the result of operative procedures dealing with the endocrines.

If a change is made in the type of metabolism of an individual after the age of growth, the measurements will change, but will change very slowly. The older the patient the more slowly the change will take place.

The nearer the measurements are to the correct figure, the more rapid will be the response to nutritional and endocrine treatment. The further the measurements are from normal, the greater the necessity for supplemental endocrine treatment along with the nutritional.

Since dental caries as well as body proportions are often the result of imperfect body chemistry, it was logical to presume that there might be some relationship between dental caries and body proportions as determined by measurements. And so a chart was made giving the body measurements and yearly rate of cavities of several hundred patients. The chart shows that the incidence of caries increases as the measurements vary from a point of about 1.420. At this point there seems to be immunity to dental caries.

It is possible to meaure a young person and, if she is subject to caries, to estimate the number of cavities which will occur in a year. This brings up another interesting observation for which no explanation is offered: namely, that when people have caries they have them at a certain yearly rate. One might possibly think that if caries are systemic in origin that the condition which promotes caries would be general throughout the mouth and that the deterioration of all teeth would coincide with the deterioration of one. However, this is not the way nature seems to have planned it. Any dentist who has practiced long enough can tell by going over his records that such and such a patient had so many cavities that year and so many the next with almost unvarying regularity. Of course, sometimes this rate will suddenly increase or decrease due to changes in environmental conditions, or for no obvious reason a susceptible person may become totally immune. Generally, changes in annual incidence of caries can be traced to changes of diet such as eating in restaurants as the result of getting a new job, going away to school, or getting married. In the case of a man, marriage changes his diet from that of his family to that of his wife's.

Many patients show immunity to caries even when their measurements are far from normal. But it is among these people that we find chronic gingivitis and pyorrhea. A series of blood tests for these people will show high phosphorus levels during part of the time covered by the tests. A series of tests may show a continued high level of phosphorus or a varying level of high and low phosphorus, but the periods of high phosphorus will occur frequently enough and be of sufficient duration to keep the density of the dentine high. It takes a continued low level of phosphorus over a period of several months to deplete the dentine of its mineral structure. The people who do have caries at a rate proportional to their measurements have a quite consistent level of phosphorus throughout the year. Therefore the amount of dental decay, the degree of disproportion in bodily measurements, and the imbalance of the calcium-phosphorus levels prove of significance to each other.

As an example of the use of one's blueprint of construction, along with complete laboratory blood and urine analysis in establishing good body chemistry, the following three typical cases are given.

A girl of fifteen was referred by a local dentist because of rampant decay and throat blisters. The latter had been present for six weeks. The patient also complained of a skin eruption on her nose which had bothered her for some years. Her body measurements when graphed indicated a deficient posterior pituitary gland. Dietary instructions and 1/100th grain of posterior pituitary were given daily and a more normal calcium-phosphorus balance was established. A report from her dentist stated that new cavities were not appearing. The skin eruption cleared up promptly. This young girl, when she first came in, was not only tall and gawky but heavy through the hips with a double curve characteristic of posterior pituitary gland deficiency. Even during the brief period when she was under treatment her figure began to change. Two years later, she was modeling clothes.

A dentist brought his thirty-year-old son in for treatment. The man had a history of dry socket every time a tooth was extracted. He was a mental case, being temporarily out of an institution under the father's care. There was no desire to add to the difficulties of the situation by incurring further dry sockets (osteomyelitis); however, extractions were necessary. His graphed measurements showed an over-active thyroid, posterior pituitary and anterior pituitary glands, to a marked degree, with a low placement of the entire graph. He was put on the natural diet plus two to three units of insulin daily to inhibit the over-activity of these glands. Within a week the patient had his first extraction. No dry sockets developed after this or following extractions. In addition, his mental condition under this treatment improved to the extent that within three months he was declared legally sane.

A young lady, twenty-one years old, of Swedish descent, averaged five to six caries yearly. Her graph showed under-activity of the thyroid, posterior pituitary and anterior pituitary glands. Her calcium-phosphorus test upheld these findings, being 10 of calcium and 2.7 of phosphorus. Because of her youth it was to be expected that her response to treatment would be rapid. Therefore it was decided to try the dietary approach alone and check the frequent calcium-phosphorus blood tests. Within two months her calcium-phosphorus test was normal. Months later, it was still the same and no new cavities had appeared and she was enjoying excellent health.

The foregoing has briefly been told to show how the measurements were developed and put into meaningful forms. Anthropologists have been measuring people for over three-fourths of a century, and the techniques they perfected and the data they collected have been valuable. This approach, however, is unique in that its object is to discover glandular heredity of an individual with the aim of establishing or maintaining good body chemistry.

II. Body Chemistry

Millions upon millions of human beings are functioning without full body efficiency. Aches and pains among mankind are far too common. Unhappiness, misery and sorrow are the pitiful results. Yet, nature did not intend man to live in such a manner. Much of this misery, in fact, practically all of it, is caused by man himself and brought upon himself. The situation can and should be different. To maintain and restore health are the goals of the medical and dental sciences, and fortunately the way to accomplish these goals is open. In the past, too much emphasis has been put upon treating symptoms (this is largely due to the demands of the patient), but to look at the problem intelligently, emphasis must be put upon treating the whole body to maintain good health throughout the life span of man.

An important way to improve health is to place the chemistry of the body in balance. Each of the billions of body cells is a chemical laboratory. Each living cell must receive nourishment; each must eliminate the waste products of cell activity. No organ or tissue of the body can function efficiently if the chemistry of cells is out of balance. Disease is body chemistry thrown out of balance—by bacterial attack, by malnutrition, by injurious physical forces, by psychic impacts and by heredity. Whatever the cause of the body's being disturbed in balance, the principle of treatment is the same—to restore the balance.

Important strides have been made in the conquest of the diseases of bacterial origin. The death rate among infants has been greatly reduced. The diseases of childhood no longer take their extravagant deathly toll. The plagues and epidemics are controlled. Pneumonia and tuberculosis have dipped to lower positions on the mortality tables. So it is with other diseases caused by bacteria.

Among zoologists and biologists in general, it is a well known fact that practically all of the higher animals (especially the mammals, of which man is one), live to an age that is five times longer than their age at maturity. There should not be an exception in the case of man and there is nothing in nature to indicate that nature made man any different in this respect. This means that man should have a natural life span of 100 years, yet few reach that age. Why? Primarily, the answer is due to what man does to his body by wearing it out long before it should be. With the understanding and scientific knowledge that is now ours, it should be possible for man to follow an intelligent course with his scientific knowledge and live to be at least a hundred—and in good health at that.

Today millions of our people are afflicted with rheumatism, diabetes, dental decay, cataracts, cancer, heart and circulatory diseases, peptic ulcers, pyorrhea and skin diseases. Most of these are conditions of degeneration. The conquest of these diseases is the most important challenge to medical science today. A Congressional Committee, making an inquiry into the toll of our major diseases— their causes, prevention and control—stated the following in their concluding report:

"There has been tremendous progress in reducing the death rate from certain diseases, particularly those of infectious nature, with a resulting increase in life expectancy. Infectious disease, for example, has diminished as a national problem because, with identification of the causes of these diseases, it has become possible to develop means of prevention, control; and when the diseases occur, their prompt and adequate treatment.

"In the case of noninfectious disease, improvement has not been marked. There has been an actual increase in the incidence of, and death rate from these diseases; especially of the chronic, degenerative diseases of an aging population.

"Adequate treatment is not now available for such afflictions as heart disease, cancer, arthritis and rheumatic dystrophy. For example, the physician knows that after an attack of coronary thrombosis or a cerebral hemorrhage he can aid the patient by treating symptoms, but cannot prevent or cure the disorder. He does not fully understand the underlying causes of these ailments and is therefore not able to eliminate them. Similarly, he may completely remove a malignant growth by surgery, or slow its growth by x-ray treatment. But if these treatments are not completely successful, as is too frequently the case, the physician is unable to do much more than to provide the palliative treatment. He does not know the cause of the tumor growth and is thus unable to truly conquer it.

"Our physicians are doing their utmost with the tools at their disposal. More and more tools are being developed. But it is no understatement to say that they do not have the knowledge they require to do a really effective job on the prevention and treatment of many chronic and degenerative diseases."

Despite these grim statements there are hopeful signs that these diseases of degeneration may be conquered. There is substantial evidence that suggests that the chemistry of the body is out of balance in every degenerative disease. There are heartening experiences that prove that when body chemistry is placed in balance some of these degenerative diseases are controlled and reversed.

One may properly ask what is the method whereby the chemistry of the body is restored to balance.

First, let us look at the human body as a kind of machine. Let us compare it to an automobile. An automobile is composed of intricate parts that work in coordination to produce energy. In addition to the mechanical parts, fuel, oil, and water are required. So long as all the parts work in unison efficiently and the quality of the fuel and oil is adequate, the automobile functions satisfactorily. If, however, one vital part fails, the automobile is no longer capable of functioning. Or if the oil or gasoline is of poor quality the automobile cannot function with satisfactory power and efficiency.

Some automobiles come off the production line with a mechanism that is not in good order. On the exterior they look like any other automobile of the same make and model. Others come off the production line in good condition, but abuse and poor care by the driver soon make them lose their power and efficiency.

To extend the analogy of the automobile and the human body, we may observe that some human beings are born with inadequate constitutions, some do not supply themselves with proper fuel in the way of foods; others misuse and abuse their bodies. A poor inborn constitution, inadequate nutrition, and unwise use of the body are causes of disease. All these causes lead to improper body chemistry and ill health.

That people often take better care of their possessions and machines than they do of their own bodies is well expressed by Alexander F. Mathias in his stimulating book entitled *The Universal Constant in Living*. In this book he states the following:

"Man is so skilled in the nature and workings of the machines he has invented, but is so very unskilled in the nature and workings of the mechanism of his own organism: he knows all about the means whereby he can keep the inanimate machines in order, and considers it his duty to make proper use of these, but he knows little or nothing about the means whereby he can keep in order that animate human machine—himself."

Everyone is familiar with the physical examination that his physician or dentist makes. He uses instruments to see and hear, to look at body parts and see them in function. He examines the urine and blood; he measures height and weight. All these tests are made to give him important information that will make the diagnosis more accurate and the treatment more effective.

The dentist or the physician who is regulating body

chemistry has a different objective, he makes a different kind of examination. He does two things: he measures the length and the circumference of the lower leg and the lower arm to receive information concerning the growth pattern and the development of the person; he takes a blood and urine sample for analysis to determine the present state of the body chemistry. These two examinations give the doctor a base-line from which to start. Because these two examinations are somewhat different from those received at the patient's usual physical examination, they should be explained in more detail.

We are all aware that people differ in body shapes and sizes. No two are exactly alike. Nor are any two personalities precisely the same. These differences in structure and personality are the result of unique forces that are exerted on each person. In large part these differences are produced by the varying amounts of chemicals produced by the glands of internal secretion (the endocrines). These glands are vital to life and well-being. When they are disordered, disease results. Diabetes and goiter are two common diseases of such origin. There are countless other conditions of disease that are produced by the disorders of the endocrine secretions.

The physical (anthropometric) measurements of the lower arm and leg give important clues to the kind of endocrine system with which a person was endowed. Some persons have a system that produces too much endocrine secretion, others too little, some more fortunate ones a well-balanced amount. Just as growth rings shown on the cross section of a tree represent the pattern of development of that tree, the human body may be measured to record the growth pattern of that person. No two trees, no two persons, are exactly alike in form, structure, or function.

Each person is endowed with a certain growth and development potential. Our ancestors are an important factor. But the development of each person is determined by the proper function and coordination of his endocrine glands. These are the regulators of all body processes. A giant is produced by too much output of the growth hormone from a part of the "master" or pituitary gland at the base of the brain. A dwarf is produced by too little output of growth hormone. There are thousands of varieties, forms, and patterns of improper function of endocrine glands between these two extremes. A cursory look at any group of people emphasizes their body differences. As their bodies differ in size and shape, they also differ in function and temperament and susceptibility to different types of disease.

After the body measurements are made, a graph (endocrinograph) is prepared by precise mathematical calculations, using a slide rule. This graph may be compared to an engineer's preliminary survey or the architect's rough drawing that is made before a bridge is erected or a house is built. This graph, unique and individual for each person, suggests the kind of physical structures with which the person began life and the degree of the efficiency of the function of these structures. It is a starting point for the appraisal of the efficiency of the body's chemistry.

After the individual graph (endocrinograph) is made, a sample of blood is taken for laboratory analysis. Blood is the essence of life. It bathes and carries nutrients to every one of the billions of cells and carries away waste products from each cell. It carries oxygen to the cells and carbon dioxide away from them. Blood transports the minerals, the vitamins and the minute hormone output from every endocrine gland. It carries the antibodies that are necessary to resist and overcome bacterial infection. Blood is the dynamic force in life. Complete blood and urine examination are done, as well as additional tests when more information is needed.

In the Page Method of regulating body chemistry the degree of efficiency of body function is expressed by the calcium-phosphorus ratio and the amount of sugar present in the circulating blood. These determinations are included in the tests made on the blood sample. The ideal toward which the method of regulation is directed is to maintain the blood sugar level at 100 milligrams, calcium

10, phosphorus 4 (or 2.5 parts of calcium to 1 part of phosphorus) per hundred cubic centimeters of blood. At these levels the body functions most successfully and efficiently in all parts and organs. To achieve these balances, small amounts of endocrine supplements are usually given while the chemistry of the body is being regulated.

To carry on life processes energy must be supplied by food. Cells and tissues that are destroyed in the life processes must be replaced by food. The quantity of food is important, but more important is its quality. Everything that the body needs in the way of food must be left out that is injurious or that the body does not need. The proper and nutritious foods are advised while the improper and harmful foods are deleted.

The diet is what is supplied in the form of food; nutrition is what the body utilizes. The diet may be satisfactory, but if the chemical processes of assimilation are not good, the nutrition is below standard. Each person has an individual capacity for food utilization. Each person must be studied separately to determine his nutritional status. The differences in persons are in large part due to their endocrine patterns.

During the course of a body chemistry audit, certain suggestions are made with respect to the types of food intake. While the study is being made some foods and drinks are prohibited. There is nothing notably harsh or difficult about these prohibitions. Many of them may be relaxed within a short time. Other food restrictions must be considered to be permanent. These will be explained to the patient as treatment progresses.

The patient must be impressed with the fact that the success of the treatment depends in large part on what he does himself. The role of the doctor is that of a director to show a patient what he may do for himself.

The degree of success in the regulation of the body's chemistry is determined by repeated blood examinations which give evidence to show if the body's chemistry is coming into balance. These blood examinations at frequent intervals record progress and the correctness or incorrectness of treatment. To achieve balance it is often necessary to change the amounts and kinds of endocrine supplements from time to time. In all cases, these endocrine products are used in minute amounts just as nature planned and produces them.

The goal of treatment is to discover the correct formula for each person. A complete study is necessary for each individual. After he has obtained the desired efficiency of his body chemistry the patient should see that it is maintained. A blood and urine examination at least once per year, at the biochemical laboratory and consultation with his doctor in person or by mail whenever the occasion demands, insures the ideal of medicine—prevention in its broadest sense.

The system of body measurements and blood analysis reveals both minor and major causes of ill health. By combining these two methods of interpretation in each case, there is considerable saving of time in arriving at a correct body chemistry formula for each person.

During the phase of study and treatment a person may feel up or down, better or worse, while his body is adjusting to a new scheme of living. This is to be expected; this is natural. These are normal swings of feeling.

The time that it will take to achieve the proper balance will be determined by the length of time it has been out of balance, by the power and vitality within the person and by the degree of cooperation from the patient.

You have the powers within yourself to improve your health. Use these powers to the fullest!

As positive proof of the effectiveness of diet and endocrine supplementation in the treatment of degenerative diseases, the following statistical example is given. Case histories of 688 patients who had come to the Page Clinic for treatment in establishing balanced body chemistry were reviewed. Each of these 688 people had ailments of various types and were seeking relief. Of the 688 only 208 had a normal blood sugar of 100 mgs. per 100 cc of blood. Blood sugar, along with calcium-phosphorus ratios and other factors of the blood, indicates the degree of normalcy of one's body chemistry. First, all of these patients were put on the basic diet which eliminates all sugar and sugar products, milk and milk products, fruit juices, coffee, alcohol and white bread for 3 days. On the basic diet alone, the number with a normal blood sugar increased to 367 out of 688. Now, you should bear in mind that these 688 patients were ill when they came seeking treatment. This indicates just how effective diet could be in maintaining health if people would follow a good, sound natural diet. All showed some improvement on the basic diet alone. The next procedure was to give each patient the minute amount of endocrine supplements needed for his or her individual needs. The results gained from basic diet, plus endocrine supplements, were remarkable. Of the 632 cases so treated, 569 attained normal blood sugar levels while the remaining 63 patients, though not attaining a normal blood sugar level, showed marked improvement. All of this statistically proves that the basis of degenerative disease lies in the functioning of the endocrine glands, and that diet is all important in influencing the endocrine glands. In short, if one has good body chemistry, he should not have degenerative diseases. Good body chemistry depends upon the endocrine glands and diet. By supplementing or inhibiting deficient glands with the amount of glandular extract needed, as worked out for a particular patient along with a sound, natural diet, good body chemistry can be attained and maintained.

One of the ideal goals of the body chemical approach to health is to reach young mothers prior to the conception of a child. Dietary correction and biochemical balance prior to conception should prepare them for a comfortable pregnancy, an uneventful birth and assure them of a normal, healthy baby. This is the true use of this work—prevention of trouble.

Many young mothers do not realize nor associate the great value of efficiency of body chemistry and correct diet with their own health and the health of their offspring. They do not realize that they prepare the way and are the donors of health to the child prior to conception and after birth. The efficiency of their body chemistry and correct diet are the determining factors as far as the health of the child is concerned. For example, it is common practice for physicians to give calcium tablets to expectant mothers. If the mother's diet is correct and her body chemistry is in good working order, she will obtain an adequate amount of calcium from her foods for herself and for the child.

It is tragic that so many young mothers are unaware of the benefits of the efficiency of body chemistry and correct diet in relation to their children. They prepare expensive layettes for the coming child, but they do not prepare their own bodies through proper diet and a top-functioning bodily mechanism for their own welfare and that of the child.

If we could provide this one service to young mothers, that of attaining and maintaining efficiency of body chemistry and following a correct diet, we would consider it a priceless contribution to the health and welfare of future generations.

Recently we received a letter from an Army Major expressing an interest in the body chemistry approach to health and requesting information concerning our work. He stated that he had four boys and wanted to give them a good start in life healthwise. We receive letters from all parts of the country from mothers who wish to learn more about improving the diet and health of their children. In our opinion, correct diet and efficiency of body chemistry are inseparable. We consider these inquiries concerning our work an encouraging sign that the parents of our nation are beginning to realize that correct diet is of major importance as far as the health of their children is concerned. If they can take the second step and learn that efficiency of body chemistry is essential, so that the body can assimilate the elements of a correct diet, then they will be on the right track. Parents are beginning to realize that the average American diet is not adequate to maintain the health of their children. Over the years it has been noted that the people who are interested in the body chemical approach to health are above average in intelligence.

Those of our patients who do not understand the methods and purpose of this approach to health fall by the wayside. The letters we receive from young parents show that our young people are intelligent, thinking individuals. Our hope and aim is to reach more of them so that they may avail themselves of the body chemistry approach to assure good health for themselves and their children.

The body chemistry approach to health can also be of value at the close of life. There are many articles appearing in the newspapers and magazines concerning the "Golden Years," the retirement years facing a vast number of our citizens today throughout the country. Some people look forward to the retirement years with pleasure and anticipation. To them they represent vistas of leisure time for the cultivation of hobbies, for making new friends, for travel and for the many things they have been unable to do because of the demands and responsibilities of home and business. Others face the retirement years with fear and misgivings. They feel that it is a time of decline, that their years of activity are ended.

The important element for the enjoyment of the retirement years, of course, is good health. With good health, the mind and body remain alert and active. The happy mind and the healthy body will look forward to the opportunity of doing new things, meeting new people, and seeing new places. There should, of course, be a slowing down of activity, but certainly not a complete halt and mental and physical deterioration.

A sensible, practical program should be worked out for eating, sleeping, work and recreation. A good diet is essential to maintain a healthy body. Good wholesome food is a must. There should be adequate physical activity but plenty of rest. There should be no extremes in either work or recreation, nor overactivity during extremes of hot or cold weather. Our bodies can take and have taken a great deal of abuse and punishment in our lifetimes, but at retirement age there should be a slowing down of pace. We should wisely recognize and accept our limitations. Especially for the elderly, the careful and proper selection of the food eaten is essential to zestful living and a good emotional attitude. The basic needs of good nutrition for the elderly do not vary much from those which apply to younger adults, but the difference is that the older person needs to pay attention to them more closely.

Doctors consider that the "geriatric years" start at the age of 40, but we all know individuals who look much younger than their years. Investigation is apt to reveal that good diet habits are largely responsible.

Dry and sallow skin, a puffy face, thick waistline, jumpy nerves, and indigestion do not equal the inevitable price one pays for being 40 or older; they equal the price one pays for incorrect dietary habits.

Many older people are vexed with diet problems. For example: In regard to so-called "health foods," the elderly person can get all the good nutrition he needs from natural foods unless advised by a physician to take food supplements.

A high protein diet is essential for the older person. His need for proteins does not decrease with increasing age.

Vitamins and minerals are as important to the diet of the older person as to the younger adult.

Generally speaking three meals a day are adequate. In some instances doctors may recommend only two. Digestion often is improved by eating three smaller meals with light in-between snacks. However, good diet is of no avail if the chemistry of the body cannot utilize the food nutrients which are taken into the stomach. Here again, efficiency of body chemistry is the determining factor for a healthy body and a sound mind both at the beginning and the close of life.

The principles expounded in this book are basic because they do not interfere with other treatments; basic because any treatment that fails to take into consideration the fundamental laws of body chemistry is inadequate; basic because even if not supplemented with any other kind of treatment, they may make it possible for the body itself to successfully undertake the restoration of health; basic because they follow the two simple rules of diet: (1)

giving the body all the materials it needs; (2) withholding the things that are injurious to it. Almost everyone can enjoy even better health and avoid the possibility of falling victim to any of the deficiency diseases by following these two simple rules of health.

When poor nutrition is thus exchanged for good, almost miraculous effects can be expected. Good body chemistry brings correct weight and its proper distribution, increased emotional stability, maximum production, heightened resistance to disease and more rapid recuperative powers.

When body chemistry is out of balance, we have body disproportions. In one type excess weight appears above the waist, in another below the waist. As the body chemistry is returned to normal, these excesses tend to be equalized. We had one case of an overweight person who lost ten pounds in two and one-half weeks although she was eating more than she had been able to eat for several years. The loss of weight was due to the returning balance of the endocrines. The improved endocrine balance was dependent upon a diet containing the essentials to the proper functioning of the glands. All the elements of nutrition were present, but special stress was laid upon vitamins and minerals as they are most likely to be deficient in our diets.

Another patient who was about normal in weight had a distinct redistribution of that weight as her body chemistry regained balance. Still other patients added to their aesthetic appeal by putting on a few pounds. But in none of these cases was there a definite program for reducing or gaining. The entire aim was to regain chemical balance of the body. With that came these other advantages.

As for emotional stability, all those who have ever been ill know that their perspective is out of focus at such times. Bring them back into body balance and their outlook on life falls into more normal channels. Healthy bodies do not germinate strong bacteria, and thus, although infectious diseases may occur in all of us at times, our resistance against them will be stronger if our body mechanisms are kept at the peak of efficiency. For example, some people become infected easily but since the pancreas is secreting ample insulin, they heal quickly. A normal person is less apt to become infected and also heals quickly. Another person, on the other hand, tends to become infected readily because the pancreas is producing an insufficient amount of insulin and heals slowly. The recuperative powers of the various types run about parallel to their capacity to heal.

It is self-evident that a chemically balanced body is more efficient than one out of balance. Therefore, in health, we can expect greater productive abilities with less fatigue than is found in a mechanism weakened by inferior parts.

In attainment of health under the body chemistry system there are two limiting factors: first, the ability of the endocrines to respond; and second, the time required for any particular endocrine pattern to return to normal. These are the limiting factors of the body chemistry approach to the degenerative diseases. The principles of this approach are based upon recognition that each individual differs from another in endocrine pattern and nutritional needs, and that in nutrition we have the means to bring about or prevent breakdown within the body.

The greatest value of this work is not in stopping the progress of disease or reversing its course but in preventing the occurrence of degenerative ills. By making regular calcium-phosphorus tests, susceptibility to these diseases can be determined before the ordinary symptoms have had an opportunity to develop. Good body chemistry can be regained through the temporary use of endocrine products and continuous adherence to proper nutrition.

The economic advantages to be gained by these health measures are considerable. Business organizations need not have the efficiency of their production limited by so many absences due to illness. The help turnover need not be so great because fewer people in a depleted physical condition need be hired. Judgments of personality and stamina will have a firmer foundation through the application of body measurement tests and the recognition of minor symptoms of good and bad body chemistry.

Good body chemistry maintained from childhood will produce human beings of physical perfection in form and line, and through proper education other qualities desirable in this field can be cultivated. Child actors and actresses of today need not continue to develop physical disproportions. Thick legs, heavy hips, bad curves at the knee, all these things can be corrected during the growing years by proper nutrition; nutrition aimed at keeping the endocrines—the determinants of growth—in proper balance.

What is needed is to apply the same standards of perfection to people that we do to farm animals and machines. The basic reason for doing so may be economic, aesthetic or a desire to see human beings give the most to life and receive from it the maximum in health and happiness. Whatever the reason, it is folly to let our civilization run itself into the ground because of failure to apply our intelligence to the preservation of a race of healthy people.

III. You and Your Glands

The secrets to the inner workings of the body chemical laboratory are the glands. The body has numerous glands such as the sweat glands and salivary glands, but the master regulators of body metabolism are the endocrine glands. They are called endocrine glands because they empty their hormones directly into the blood stream. The blood stream then takes these hormones, which are chemical compounds manufactured in minute amounts, to the rest of the body and other glands. The glands work in harmony or unison. If one is malfunctioning, it will affect the others to a greater or lesser degree. Our endocrine glands not only take part in everything that we do, but actually make it possible for us to do what we do. They govern our temperament and, physiologically, our everyday activities. For example, lift your little toe or finger; it is vital hormones that see to it that blood sugar is in the blood stream to feed the muscles so that muscle power is available. Cut your hand, or any part of your body, and hormones help to control inflammation and keep infection from setting in. These hormones may be described as tiny hydrogen bombs which are powerful almost beyond description. They circulate through the blood system, going to the right places and doing just the right things in a normally healthy body. But, when one group of hormones are in excess, deficient, or otherwise abnormal, they upset the entire glandular system with the result that the entire body mechanism and functions are out of order.

There are eight of the endocrine glands which taken all together weigh only approximately two ounces. Yet, this is probably the most important two ounces in the entire body. These glands function as a board of directors, council of ministers, and regulators of body chemistry. They work together, in a healthy situation, so harmoniously that if one is sluggish, another gives it a helping hand or can assume part of its function depending upon the circumstances. They are further subdivided into working groups. One of these functional groups consists of the pineal-thymus sex glands. Similar functional group relations exist between the pituitary, thyroid and adrenal glands which are functionally connected with the sex glands. To understand these glands and their functions, it is necessary to take up each one separately.

The pituitary gland has been termed the most remarkable component of the human body because of its great influence on the other glands and may be said to be likened to the conductor of a symphony orchestra in reference to its relationship to the other glands. The pituitary is a double organ, the anterior pituitary and the posterior pituitary, which are separate glands. Together these two lobes are about the size of a large pea situated in the bony cavern on the underside of the brain at about the center of the head. The position of the pituitary gland, which gives it maximum protection, is indicative of its importance.

One of the most fascinating substances produced by the anterior pituitary gland is the growth hormone. It controls growth. An under-active anterior pituitary gland may not produce enough of this hormone for the individual to reach the maximum height to which he would ordinarily grow, and is responsible for dwarfism. Man has created some dwarfs purposely by inbreeding for very under-active anterior pituitary glands. An example of this is the dachschund dog which owes its dwarfed form to a considerable under-active anterior pituitary gland.

Conversely, if the anterior pituitary gland is very much over-active in its production of the growth hormone, the result is a giant. Most circus giants are a result of a very abnormal over-activity. If the anterior pituitary gland grows larger in adult life, after one's skeleton has become set, parts of the skeleton may begin to grow again. Since the growth zones have become completely set, only the free ends of the bones of the chin, feet, nose, and hands can grow. This disease is known as acromegaly. It is the growth hormone from the anterior pituitary which prompts growth in a new born babe; it receives these human growth hormones from its mother's milk. Those who drink cow's milk get the cow growth hormone. That is why those who have an over-active anterior pituitary gland should not have milk after the weaning period. More will be said about this in the chapter on milk. An over-active anterior pituitary gland is often associated with cancer. It is easy to see this relationship when we realize that most of the types of cancer are really cells gone wild in their growth pattern. When the gland is over-active it is producing too much of the powerful growth hormone and it is bound to have its effect upon the other glands of the body and the cells. The importance of this gland can hardly be overly exaggerated when we realize that the anterior pituitary may be described as a kind of governor of all the other endocrine glands.

The pituitary gland plays a major part in the birth process. Following delivery of a baby it releases a very minute amount of a hormone which causes contraction of the mother's womb. This is one of nature's guards against excessive bleeding that can result in death. A few days following birth another hormone from the anterior pituitary, is released. It is one of the truly extra-ordinary chemicals ever discovered—prolactin—which stimulates the breast to produce milk and largely accounts for mother love. To judge from experimentation with animals, it seems most likely that individuals' ability to produce this hormone is responsible for their differing abilities to nurse babies and also in their attitude toward babies. All have observed that some women become natural mothers while others, if they perform their duties as good mothers, do it mainly because of social pressure.

The pituitary gland, along with the sex glands and the adrenal cortex, also plays quite an important part in sex.

There certainly is no doubt that sex behavior is subject to all kinds of environmental influences, but to one who is familiar with endocrinology and biological variability, there is also no doubt that the glandular system, which is distinctive in each person, plays a major part in sex variability.

Another substance produced by the anterior pituitary is ACTH, the adrenocorticotropic hormone. It seems that this hormone has to do with disposition or general feeling of well-being. This indicates definitely that the hormonal differences of individuals may have a great deal to do with people's dispositions.

The posterior pituitary gland secretes hormones which help to control the salt and water balance of the body and control the gravity or density of the urine. If it were not for this control an individual would urinate as much as three gallons or more of urine a day.

When the posterior pituitary gland is not functioning properly one may be quite prone to diabetes insipidus, (excessive urination), arthritis, pyorrhea, high blood pressure, and other degenerative diseases depending upon how such a dysfunction affects the other glands and the body as a whole. An under-active posterior pituitary may be the reason for sterility in women.

From this little survey of the function of the pituitary gland it is easy to see that it is very complicated in both structure and function. The various parts manufacture many different hormones which themselves then interact with the other glands of the body in carrying out their special functions. As pointed out previously, these hormones are carried to all parts of the body through and by the blood stream. That is why the blood analysis is so important in any approach to body chemistry.

To a very considerable degree, our general well-being is dependent upon the speed at which our bodies live. The rate of speed of the basic cellular bodily processes is regulated by the thyroid gland. This gland is butterfly shaped and straddles the windpipe. It is approximately the size of a walnut. However, its size is dependent on many factors such as heredity, which determines whether or not it is normal or abnormal to begin with, and environment such as diet, which can greatly affect it. The thyroid gland has been likened to the accelerator of a car because it speeds up or slows down our body activities. The thyroid hormone determines whether the rate at which we live is in a slow, sluggish, sleepy, half-alive world or in an energy-charged, racing one. The hormonal production of a normal thyroid is only one twenty-eight-hundredths of an ounce per day (1/2800). When the gland produces too much hormone, that person is then said to have an over-active thyroid (hyperthyroidism) and when it produces too little, the individual has an under-active thyroid gland (hypothyroidism). When the gland is under-active it can cause the metabolism to slow down to such a subnormal level that the person may be said to be merely vegetating in his existence. When a person is suffering from an over-active thyroid gland, he is always in a rush and is the type that may be described as "burning the candle at both ends." Either one of these abnormal conditions, particularly when they become acute, can cause devastation to both body and mind. When one has an over-active thyroid, some of the symptoms which may be present are a ravenous appetite, pounding heart, and high blood pressure, and is likely to be very susceptible to ulcers and heart ailments associated with the nerves that control the heart.

With advancing age the thyroid often gradually tapers off its production of vital thyroid hormone. That is why many elderly people are said to have become cold natured in their advancing years. In these cases their bodies just are not producing enough heat. Sterility in some women is also due to an under-active thyroid which has slowed their bodily activities to such a degree that they are sterile.

The most commonly known disease of the thyroid gland is goiter. This is just one of a number of degenerative diseases which may afflict it. Goiter may be associated with either an over-active thyroid or an under-active one. One of the major causes of goiter is due to a dietary deficiency of the mineral iodine. Iodine is extensively distributed in nature, but there are some parts of the world in which it is not present. People in these parts may suffer from an iodine deficiency. The natural way in which the body gets its iodine is from food, and sea foods.

An adult requires only 15 billionths of an ounce of iodine per day, but even that minute amount is not available in areas where iodine is deficient in the water, soil and plants, and therefore in the diet. An example of such areas are the Alps Mountain Regions of Europe and our own middle western states around the Great Lakes region. Today inorganic iodine is added to our table salt to guard against this deficiency. However, it is much healthier for the body to get its iodine in the natural form from foods. A healthy thyroid gland contains about four ten-thousandths (4/10,000) of an ounce of iodine. Other types of goiter are caused by other factors and have nothing to do with iodine.

Dr. Roger Williams, the outstanding biochemist of the University of Texas, who discovered one of the B vitamins, has stated that there are a great many people who are somewhat deficient in thyroid hormone and that they would be greatly benefited by taking a minute amount of it orally. However, these people do not usually feel sick enough to go to the doctor, so nothing is done about the situation. Still, it must be born in mind that the dosage must be minute and prescribed according to the individual patient's needs. Too much is just as harmful as too little.

The hormone manufactured by the thyroid gland is transported to the cells in a state of loose chemical combination with the globulin fraction of the proteins in the blood stream. In this condition the hormone can be taken from the blood for measurements of protein-bound iodine, which is generally referred to simply as a PBI blood test. This test is one of the most reliable for determining the amount of thyroid hormone circulating in the blood stream. In a normal person there should be a concentration of five to seven micrograms of protein-bound iodine per 100 cubic centimeters of blood, or five to seven parts per

100 million. When the thyroid is over-active the concentration often rises to 10 to 20 micrograms, whereas with an under-active thyroid it may go down to less than one microgram. The PBI test is one of the many tests used in our thorough and extensive blood analyses in determining the condition of one's body chemistry.

The parathyroids, four little glands about the size of little wheat grains, are situated alongside the thyroid. The main function of the hormone produced by the parathyroids is that of regulating the blood calcium level. They determine the transport of calcium from the bones into the bloodstream, body tissues, and see that excess calcium is thrown out in the urine. The calcium we get through our food, is first deposited in the bones (this is also controlled by other hormones) and later taken to the blood as the body requires. Of course, the parathyroids are in turn largely regulated by the other glands, but when the parathyroid hormone is deficient or lacking the body does not have enough calcium. One disease associated with calcium deficiency is pyorrhea; another is tetany, a condition in which the muscles twitch and spasms often appear. Calcium also inhibits the neuromuscular irritability of the body tissues. When there is too much calcium in the body it may result in arthritic deposits, kidney stones, and cataracts. How the calcium is utilized depends upon one's body chemistry.

The adrenals are little yellowish-brown glands which sit atop the kidney. We can get something of their importance when it is realized that each minute they receive six times their own weight in blood. The adrenals consist of two major parts and may be likened to a walnut. The kernel, which consists of nerve cells, is called the medulla, and the shell is called the cortex. These two parts of the adrenal glands produce remarkable and very powerful hormones.

Adrenalin is secreted by the kernel of the adrenals. Due to its part in preparing us for emergencies, adrenalin may be termed the "fight or flee" hormone. For example, a man who himself has been injured, rushes into a burning house and rushes out carrying the refrigerator, and then collapses. It was adrenalin that provided such a great spurt of power and strength. In times of great stress or danger, the hormonal production of adrenalin may suddenly shoot up to ten times the normal level, with the result that the heart and breathing rates increase while the level of energizing blood sugar shoots up. The normal level of adrenalin in the blood stream ranges from one two-billionth to two one-billionths, so you can see that it takes only the tiniest amount, even for the greatest emergencies. In that the adrenals cannot be sure how a conflict will come out, they also greatly quicken the clotting time of blood so as to reduce the loss of blood if one is cut. It is also adrenalin that acts as an oxidative ferment during nerve-cell activity, dilates the pupils of the eyes, contracts the capillaries, raises blood pressure, mobilizes sugar from the liver, increases the tonus of the heart muscles, and seems to play some part in the formation of skin pigmentation.

The adrenal cortex, the shell of the adrenals, manufactures a large number of different hormones or hormonelike chemicals; at present some 28 have been identified of which one is a sex hormone. Some of the body functions influenced by the adrenal cortex are mineral levels in the blood stream, carbohydrate metabolism, kidney function, the ability of muscles to respond to stimulation, stimulation of the sex glands, and resistance to stress caused by such things as bacterial poisons, too much insulin and thyroid hormone. Now substances similar to the adrenal cortex hormone are produced synthetically, such as cortisone. These were at first hailed as wonder cures for arthritis and many other diseases, but their use in very large doses has also proven to be something of a curse. Once again it is reiterated that too much of the endocrine hormones are just as bad as too little. In most all of the cases that I have seen, the patient would have been much better off to have never taken cortisone.

Little is known about the pineal and thymus glands. The pineal gland may restrain the action of the sex glands while the thymus seems to play a part in the maturing process from childhood to adulthood. When adulthood has been reached, the thymus dries up and shrinks to only a small part of its former size.

The isles of Langerhans of the pancreas produce insulin. When insulin is not produced, the disease of diabetes is present. This is known as hypoinsulinism. People can be born with this condition or a tendency for it or it may develop due to the use of too much sugar. Insulin is carried by the blood stream to the muscles and the liver, whereby these organs are then able to utilize the sugar in the blood and to store it in the form of glycogen. Many people suffer from an under-active production of insulin, but unfortunately they do not recognize such until the situation has manifested itself seriously.

However, too much insulin is also very harmful. When the pancreas produces too much insulin, the condition is referred to as hyperinsulinism. Too much insulin in the system produces a low blood sugar. This is shown in the following symptoms: fainting or dizzy spells, ravenous appetite and general weakness. Whenever there is over-production of insulin it may be accompanied by an under-production of the anterior pituitary gland, the opponent of the isles of Langerhans. The anterior pituitary produces hormones which convert glycogen (stored body sugar) to usable sugar and puts it into the blood stream. One of the most important functions of insulin is that of fighting infection. Quite often people who constantly suffer from one type of infection or another suffer from having too little insulin. Insulin plays many parts other than in just preventing diabetes, but most people only associate its use with diabetes. A minute dosage of insulin is often all that many patients need to get their body chemistry functioning to its normal healthy level. It should be added also that a faulty diet, particularly sugar, is one of the foods which is definitely injurious to the insulin producing pancreas.

The sex glands are exceptionally important because they produce vital hormones which are necessary for a balanced body chemistry. The male sex glands, known as testes, produce the male hormone testosterone. This is an androgen. Both males and females need this hormone, but naturally men produce more than the female—it is the so-called masculine hormone. When a person produces too much androgen, that individual is characterized as being andric—in other words too male from the hormonal or glandular viewpoint. This is manifest in personality also; andrics are go-getters, they drive themselves too much, just as do those with an over-active thyroid. One sign of andricity is baldness, and andrics are likely to be much more subject to ulcers, cancer, heart or circulatory. diseases. Andric men are especially prone to have prostate gland trouble.

The female sex glands, termed ovaries, produce the hormone estrogen in extremely minute quantities. During a woman's 30 childbearing years, she produces an amount of estrogen hormones approximately the weight of a postage stamp. At the time of puberty it takes only a very minute amount of estrogen to bring about such a change, the amount being approximately equal to only one little corner of a postage stamp. Individuals producing too much estrogen are termed gynics. Gynics are usually more of a submissive type of person. In order to be normal and healthy, men also must have a very minute amount of estrogen. Not enough estrogen may result in rendering one more susceptible to heart and circulatory diseases, nervous disorders, and mental disturbances. However, too much is also very harmful.

The term gynic is used to designate the condition of over-production of estrogen while the term andric is employed for the condition of over-production of testosterone or progesterone. In using the terms andricity and gynicity, it should be pointed out that this in no way has to do with sexual perversion or homosexuality. It refers to the production and function of the sex hormones in the human body Each individual must have the proper balance of them to have good body chemistry and good health. Men and women must have a certain amount of both male and female hormones; naturally each sex requires more of its own sex hormone than that of the opposite sex, but both must be present in the proper amount to insure that the glands function properly. So, when it is said that a woman is andric, it does not mean that she is masculine. It merely means that she has an over-producing of androgens and is thus in an unhealthy situation, manifesting personality traits, which may make it very difficult for her to get along with her husband, if he is also andric. Likewise, when a man is gynic it does not mean that he is feminine, but that he has too high a production of estrogen and is thus likely to have a slower metabolism than normal, which also presents itself in personality or disposition. Two gynics of opposite sex are not apt to get along together very well either. However, when an andric and gynic marry they usually get along very well, particularly during the childbearing period. Nature has that way of taking care of future generations. In this case with an andric and gynic marrying, both of whom are abnormal in their andric-gynic balance, nature plays its part by seeing that at least a certain percentage of the children from this marriage will have a chance of being born with normal glandular patterns. You often hear it said that opposites attract, and this is one of the explanations for that. Of course, the ideal is for two people to both have perfect glandular balance. This is where your blueprint of construction comes in; it tells the story. Now, it does not mean that the situation is hopeless. By taking glandular supplement and following the diet along with understanding of the problem, the parties concerned can be made compatible.

In this approach to good health, it is easy to see what is done when a gland is under-active. You merely give the proper amount of that gland's hormone to the patient. But, what about the gland that is over-active. We have two divisions of the glandular system, the build-up glands, which are isles of Langerhans of the pancreas, posterior pituitary, parathyroid and adrenal cortex and female hormone, and the breakdown glands, which are made up of the thyroid, anterior pituitary, adrenal medulla and andric hormones. These two sets of glands are opposed to each other. For example, when the thyroid is over-active, the secretion from the pancreas may lower it. In other words each gland has its opposite or opposites which will inhibit its action. When the glands are functioning normally, glandular balance has been established. Glandular imbalance lies at the root of most, if not all, degenerative diseases.

Your blueprint of construction tells the glandular pattern with which you were born, but it does not tell what has happened to your glands since you were born. Thus further diagnosis becomes necessary and the tools here are extensive blood analysis, urine analysis, and blood pressure readings. As you have seen above, it is the blood that carries the glandular hormones to the various parts of the body and it is hormones themselves which determine the constituency of the blood.

All the tests are exceptionally important, but the major ones for a general index to efficiency of body chemistry are the calcium-phosphorus and blood sugar levels. During my 40 years of practice and research with many thousands of cases, it has been determined that the proper level of calcium-phosphorus is two and one-half parts calcium to one part phosphorus. The blood sugar level should be exactly 100 milligrams of blood sugar per 100 cubic centimeters of blood. The endocrine glands which participate in one way or another upon blood sugar levels are the isles of Langerhans of the pancreas, anterior pituitary, adrenals, the thyroid and the sex glands. From all this you can see that there is a complicated process of inter-action of these glands. For example, over-activity of the anterior pituitary may lead to a high blood sugar level, whereas under-activity of the isles of Langerhans can produce the same effect. Low or high blood sugar levels in turn affect the calcium-phosphorus level of the blood. We have already seen what the effects of too much or too little calcium may be. Excessive phosphorus is also dangerous, it may cause headaches, nausea, yellow skin, weariness, and inflammatory conditions which may show up anywhere in the body. Certainly when the cholesterol level is too high the glands are not working properly. The cholesterol level actually has little to do with diet but is dependent upon proper glandular functions and is only indirectly influenced by diet as such influences the glands. Too high or too low a cell volume informs the doctor that something is wrong, and so it goes with each one of the analyses made.

It cannot be emphasized too much that the use of endocrine hormones in treatment to bring about good body chemistry must be used in very minute amounts which vary with each patient.

In dealing with people, no two of whom are indentical, each person must be dealt with as an individual. One cannot prescribe that everyone suffering from a specific degenerative disease, such as heart attacks, should receive the same amount of the same hormone or even the same treatment. The dosage that is just right for one person may be undesirable for another, but when used in the proper amount the results are as desired. Hormones keep our bodies functioning properly, or improperly, depending upon whether or not glandular balance is present. The body chemistry approach is to establish what is needed for each individual for his specific needs. In other words, the body chemistry approach to good health treats the whole person as an individual, not just the disease. When good body chemistry has been established, and is maintained, there should be no premature degeneration. With maximum chemical efficiency each individual should then be expected to live the whole life span with which he was endowed by God and nature in a normal healthy state of well-being.

IV. Diet and Nutrition

Among the numerous changes brought about by civilization within the modern era, none is more profound or of greater importance than that in the realm of man's diet. Many of these changes have been good and even necessary due to the large concentration of people in cities. Unfortunately, many of these changes have been detrimental to the health oi man and no doubt account for many of the illnesses that are associated with modern living. Within the area of diet and nutrition so much misinformation is dispensed that it is difficult for one to know the truth. There are natural laws which govern diet and nutrition, just as natural laws govern everything else in nature. Man is a creature oi natural law, and he must follow it. The penalty for disobeying the laws of nature are poor health, degenerative diseases, and eventual extinction.

Many people think that diet and nutrition are synonymous; however, they mean different things. Nutrition is dependent partially upon diet, in that it is through diet that the body is supplied with food for assimilation to feed and nourish the cells. In other words, man does not live on what he eats, but rathei on what his body digests and assimilates. The body is not nourished by what we swallow, but by what passes through the villi of the intestinal canal into the blood. Naturally, an inadequate or deficient diet dooms one to poor and deficient nutrition. A good, wholesome diet is always recommended, but it does not always provide for good nutrition. Sometimes the body cannot assimilate it. Body assimilation of food depends upon the functioning of the endocrine and exocrine glands. If the glands are functioning improperly, the result is poor nutrition. Many people are born with faulty glandular mechanisms, and thus are described, quite often, as sickly or puny children. However, in the vast majority of cases, a good and proper natural diet will at least help improve, and perhaps cure in some cases, a faulty endocrine system. A poor diet is always injurious to a greater or lesser degree, depending upon the heredity of the individual and the functioning of the endocrine glands.

If we study a schematic drawing which represents man's progress during the last million years, we find that we know very little about him any further back than ten thousand years. There may have been many civilizations prior to ten thousand years ago, but if they existed, no evidence of them remains. Man's works do not last long due to upheavals of nature, deposits of sand, silt and water, and the wearing away of mountains and the fillings of the seas. But within the last ten thousand years we know that our ancestors were very primitive. They lived much like any other animals. They ate what nature provided, in the way it was provided for the most part. They were guided in what they ate by their opportunity to get food. They selected what tasted good to them when they had a choice. They drank water. The point is that they survived to carry on, otherwise, we would not be here.

Only a short time ago, less than five hundred years for most of our ancestors, man began to greatly develop his mechanical ability, which already made him unique among animals. By speech, and later writing, he was able to build upon the discoveries of his progenitors. This amounted to a revolution in his habits and mode of living. This revolution gained momentum with every generation, until we find that man in the last few generations has done more technologically than all previous generations together.

This technological progress has been so rapid that we have left our tried-and-true customs of living behind. We have little background of experience to guide us. Our tendency is to discard customs of the past. They have become "old fashioned." We have adopted new things without trial of time, from antibiotics to foods manufactured to taste good, or to please the eye. We have corrupted our tastes to the extent that natural foods have less appeal for us. We drink, not because of thirst, but because of taste, or for the effect it will have upon our nervous systems. We welcome the new; we discard the old.

This revolution in technology is aided and abetted by commercial interests. We have learned that people accept as true almost any statement if it is repeated often enough. Very few people like to think or to analyze. Success in life is measured by most people in the amount of money accumulated, not how it was done, providing, of course, it was legal. Seldom a thought is given as to the good or harm a manufactured food product may produce.

We read history not so much to guide us, but for the interest it produces. Instead of profiting by what we learn from the past, we have to learn the hard way by repeating the failures which history might teach us to avoid.

Our mechanical age has given us many valuable conveniences, but when we include food processing in our achievements, we have ignored what these innovations do to our bodies. We do not realize that our physiology has not changed, that our bodies work in the same way they always did, and that foods must be used that fit the demands of our bodies.

Modern man has come to regard eating as important only in so far as it satisfies his hunger or gluttony. He forgets that man is an integral part of nature. The present day human being has largely been formed by the diet of the first men, millions of years ago, and there has been no great changes in form since. The workings of his digestion system are not significantly different from those of most higher animals. Man should realize that he does not have the right to arbitrarily violate the laws of nature; to do so results in degenerative diseases for himself, and poor heredity for his children and grandchildren.

Man lives on three types of basic raw materials: these are carbohydrates, fats, and proteins. Good health demands that a person have a proper balance of these from wholesome sources.

Carbohydrates provide the primary source of bodily energy which maintains body temperature and activity; they also provide some of the building materials for body tissue. Carbohydrates are supplied by vegetables, fruits and starches; these include bread, grains, potatoes, beans, tubers, legumes, and berries, to mention only a few. In the modern world, due to the so-called ingenuity of man, carbohydrates also include processed or refined unnatural foods such as white bread, sugar, and polished white rice. Carbohydrates do more than just supply the raw materials for energy, they also supply vital minerals, vitamins and enzymes which are necessary for proper nutrition. Today, largely for economic reasons, and because of the acquired and cultivated taste of man, humans have become more and more carbohydrate eaters, and within the last century or less, excessive eaters of refined carbohydrates. Instead of being first and foremost a hunter, man has become an agrarian, raising his primary food materials in the form of grains and vegetables. Years ago these crops were raised on virgin soil, generally rich in the natural mineral nutrients so necessary to bodily health. Today, much of man's food, in fact practically all of it, is grown extensively on soil that must be replenished with commercial fertilizers. Much of this food lacks the mineral and vitamin content that should be present. Then it is even robbed more through refining and commercial preparation, so that it has more eye appeal, but less nutritive value. The two best examples of this are refined sugar and white flour which may be described as "empty calories" because they lack all of the vitamins and minerals necessary to sustain health. Sugar, sucrose to be exact, has been so prepared that it is too refined for the body mechanism to handle in a normal manner with ease. So injurious is it to the body that a special chapter is devoted to the harmful effects of sugar on the body.

The diet should contain enough carbohydrates to insure

enough calories necessary to carry out body processes and energy for bodily activity, including the functioning of muscles and nerves. Carbohydrates are the major fuel of the body, and the energy they supply is very important in building body structures from other raw materials. The body stores carbohydrates in the form of glycogen. It is carbohydrates from which body fat is built. L one wishes to lose weight he should curtail or eliminate the starchy carbohydrates, particularly bread and grains, from his diet.

Fats are necessary in the diet in that they supply essential unsaturated fatty acids, carry certain vitamins, and provide reserve fuel for the body. Fat may be described as a secondary storage fuel of the body. There are two major sources of fat—animal and vegetable. We are all familiar with lard, cream, and butter, which are animal fats. Vegetable oils include safflower oil, peanut oil, corn oil, and a host of others. Specific unsaturated fatty acids are necessary for healthy cell structure. Fat serves as a source or carrier of the fat-soluble essential vitamins, such as A, D, and E. Fat is the most concentrated fuel food and should be included in the diet more than it is. Fat does not produce fat to any significant degree as is erroneously believed by most people. It is the carbohydrates—starches and sugar—that produce fat; usually obesity s the result of not only a faulty diet but also malfunctioning body chemistry as well. Fat is necessary for the production of bile, which is essential to proper digestion and elimination. The lack of enough fat in the diet accounts for constipation in many cases.

There are some fats which are harmful to good health. As might be suspected, these are the fats which have been tampered with by man to make for better eye appeal or easier handling. These are the saturated or hydrogenated fats such as margarine, vegetable shortenings, and hydrogenated peanut butter. In their natural state, these fats are perfectly good, but when they are hydrogenated they are put in a state that the human body is not equipped to handle easily. When a vegetable oil is hydrogenated, it means that hydrogen has been run through it and that atoms of hydrogen have combined with natural molecules thus making the oil a smooth solid when cool. This is fine for the palate and economy, but not good for your health. Fat is one thing which a person is not likely to eat too much of, particularly animal fat. When one has had enough fat he can hardly eat more and will become nauseated by over-indulgence.

Whenever eating meat—chops, steaks, roast, etc.—one would be wise to eat part of the fat, as it is essential to good health. Too often we turn up our noses at the fat, and thus waste the part that is of prime importance for balanced nutrition.

Protein is necessary because it provides vital amino acids which the body must have for growth and mainte-nance of tissues. There are eight protein constituents, all belonging to the class of amino acids, that are required in the diet to maintain, repair, and build body tissue. There are at least twelve, and perhaps more, additional ones that are made in the body through combining fragments of protein and carbohydrate. There is no single food that provides all the types of amino acids required by the body in the right proportions, with the exception of the fresh meat and fat in the proper proportions. Just about every-thing in the body consists of protein, and thus its value cannot be overestimated. A good analogy is to state that we consist of protein in the same respect that a car con-sists of metal. Protein is arranged in one way to form bone, brain cells, and tissue, while in a car, metal is used to form the doors, body, engine, and wheels.

There are two major kinds and sources of protein: ani-mal and plant. Animal protein consists of meat, fish, fowl, eggs, and milk. For man, animal protein is the best be-cause it closely resembles human protein in structure, and can be more readily and completely assimilated by the body. Also, animal protein contains mineral salts and vita-mins along with valuable blood pigment. Of all the foods that man eats, animal protein requires the least amount of work for digestion and is the easiest to assimilate. Animal protein leaves only a minute residue in comparison with carbohydrates.

Vegetable protein is also important and is found in largest quantities in whole grains, seeds, beans, legumes, peas, nuts, etc. Vegetable protein alone cannot sustain healthy life because it does not contain enough of all of the amino acids that are essential. There is only one plant that can be classed as a complete protein—the soy bean, but it is so low in two of the essential amino acids that it cannot serve as a complete protein for human consumption. In fact, most all plants lack methionine, one of the essential amino acids. Vegetable protein, when supplemented properly by animal protein, makes an excellent combination. Health cannot be maintained on a diet that omits animal protein.

One will immediately ask about vegetarians. On close examination it will be found that vegetarians omit meat from their diet, but include milk, cheese, dairy products, and eggs—all animal protein. Milk is a form of modified blood, more specifically it may be termed white blood. The white of an egg, which is better for the body when cooked, is 100 per cent protein. It is necessary for a vegetarian to eat a relatively large amount of food in order to meet his basic needs because plant foods, due to their high cellulose content, are not easily assimilated and necessitate more work in chewing, flow of digestive juices, and intestinal movement. As far as the human body is concerned, vegetable protein is a poor substitute for animal protein.

Actually the digestive mechanism of man is adapted to a mixed meat and vegetable diet. Human teeth consist of three types: canines or piercing teeth of the meat-eating animals, the incisors of plant-eating animals, and the molars or grinders of grain and nut-eating animals. With respect to structure, human teeth are conclusive proof that the human body is adapted to a mixed animal and plant diet. Man has specific digestive ferments for meat proteins, and other special digestive juices for carbohydrates. His stomach and intestinal tract is equipped to handle both.

Man is naturally adapted to a mixed diet of animal and plant foods.

There are specific elementary laws of nutrition that apply to man and from which there is no escape. One of these laws is that we get our energy, measured in calories, from the food we eat and we cannot get more energy out of a given food than it contains. Another law is that in addition to calories we must have other nutrients such as minerals and vitamins. No diet can supply the raw materials for good health if it lacks even a single one of these numerous essential elements. Another law is that diet must not contain any harmful things. Only a few decades ago, there was practically no problem with foods containing things harmful to the body. Today this has become a crucial problem. Practically all of the foods that we buy in the markets contain chemicals added by man. Some of these chemicals are known to be especially harmful and a host of others are probably equally harmful. Have you realized that most of the food that you buy comes from chemically treated seeds, planted in chemically treated soil, saturated with chemical poisons to kill insects, refined and processed with a huge number of chemical additives and preservatives of one type or another, and finally packaged or canned with chemical contaminants? The public generally believes that it is fully protected by the food laws, but there are so many inadequacies and legal loopholes that the public is most inadequately protected. It is not known how many chemicals now being put into foods may be capable of inducing cancer. It is true that a small amount of most chemical preservatives, and pesticides, cannot be shown to be harmful to the body, but just because a minute amount cannot be proven to be harmful is no sign that it actually is not. Many of these chemicals, which are actually poisons, have a cumulative effect, that is, they accumulate in the body and only after years of use will the harmful effects become apparent.

Whenever you buy cereals, packaged goods, or canned goods in the store, read the labels carefully to see what chemical preservatives have been added. They have long chemical names, so naturally only a chemist understands exactly what they are, while others are merely listed as food additives. My advice is to leave them alone. Even so, you are getting some due to the insecticides, etc., used on vegetables and fruits. Fruits and vegetables should be washed thoroughly to get as much of the residue removed as is possible. Anyone who wishes to explore this topic further should read *The Poisons in Your Food* by William Longgood, which was recently published.

The Food and Drug Administration is finally becoming aware of the fact that these things are true. They are banning the use of certain insecticides and sweeteners. They have been asked to test more than six hundred food additives now in general use.

The means of estimating the dietary needs of each individual are twofold: heredity and natural needs, which, for convenience may be termed instincts.

First, physical characteristics indicate ancestry. In the past, people in general did not move about much; they lived and died in the same place and so did their children from one generation to another. As the generations went on, their physical characteristics were modified by their particular environment. Nutrition, an important part of their environment, was reflected in their bodily developments in as much as those who were best suited to the foods of certain areas survived and reproduced.

On the northern coasts were the Nordics. They were mainly fishermen and hunters and ate very few vegetables. Their chief source of food was fish and consequently their bodies became adapted to a high mineral intake. Their descendants are distinguished by fair skin and blue eyes. They are meat and fish eaters with a digestive system suitable to the handling of these foods. In this type of person, digestive ills can often be traced to the stretching of the stomach by the consumption of a very high carbohydrate diet—a diet to which their digestive tract is not adapted.

The Mediterranean peoples had a diet of animal foods and grain. These foods in their natural state, unrefined or devitalized by improper preparation, contained the minerals and vitamins necessary to growth and health, but not in the same quantities as the fish diet of the Nordics. Therefore, their bodies adapted themselves to a lesser amount of minerals, and their physiques were different. Among them, round heads and dark eyes are the rule. They are accustomed to a high carbohydrate intake and have digestive tracts which are suitable for the handling of this type of food.

Due to migration and improved facilities of transportation, we find today not only Nordics and Mediterraneans, but many mixtures in our country. In these people of mixed racial stock, the predominating factor is registered in their physical appearance and largely indicates their dietary requirement.

The second means of determining the dietary needs of each individual are the instincts. We all marvel at the efficiency of instinct in animals, the instinct that directs the birds to go south before winter comes; that leads the bear to fatten himself and dig a hole for the hibernation period; the instincts that make for the survival and reproduction of wild life. We marvel at these things and then cover up our own instincts with social laws and a veneer of civilization and habits. Why not use our intelligence, and instead of fighting our instincts, let them work for us; why not consider our instincts as tools to be used? When your body needs water it tells you so through a sense of thirst. You put a glass of water to your lips and drink. You stop. Who told you to stop? A mechanism inside you suddenly signaled, "enough." If you trust your body to tell you when you have had enough water even before that water has entered your stomach, why can't you trust it to tell you other things which it needs and how much it should have? This your instinct will do if it has not been dulled by the use of drugs or refined foods. It is my belief that a person will not need to consider the number of calories in his diet, the amount of energy foods and so forth, if an adequate supply of minerals is provided and devitalized foods are omitted.

The amounts and kinds of foods required by a given individual will be determined by his natural make-up and tastes. Today, children hardly have the opportunity to know their natural "instincts" for wholesome food. As soon as they are born they are given a special formula in milk; then specially prepared, chemically preserved, refined baby foods. As they grow older they are given refined grains, white bread, cake, candy, and a host of other empty calories as well as processed foods of all descriptions. It is a crime, because they are never given the opportunity to know what natural, wholesome food is, and their abilities to taste are warped to such an extent that when they have the opportunity to experience natural foods, they think them strange and unnatural. Fortunately, the body can respond to what is right very rapidly, and usually, when one dispenses with refined, commercially prepared foods, he regains his ability to enjoy the naturally wholesome flavor of good food intended by nature within a few weeks.

In a state of nature we have four tastes—sweet, sour, salt, and bitter. Poisonous foods are generally bitter, and so this is chiefly a protective taste. Sweet, sour and salt lead us to a variety of foods. In no one of them, for example honey or lemons, do we find just one nutritional element; each contains vitamins, proteins, and carbohydrates. So when our bodies crave sweet or sour they are demanding not an unadulterated sweet, like sugar, but sweet plus. And generally it is the plus which is of the greater importance to our physical well-being. We need to use our intelligence in our physical well-being. We need to use our intelligence in our selection of food and remember that much of the chemistry of foods is still unknown. We must consider our dietary needs on the basis of what natural foods have proven useful in survival. By adding that to our chemical knowledge, our means of transmitting ideas and transporting foods, we should be able to maintain a general standard of health and efficiency far and above anything known in history. After all, it is stupid for civilized peoples to demand mechanical perfection and efficiency of machines, and yet so neglect their own body mechanisms that they are always running under par, or being sent to the workshop for repairs.

An experiment in child feeding would seem to substantiate faith in the ability of human instincts to still be effective in food selection. Sixteen children in Chicago, who showed evidence of rickets and/or dental decay, were given their choice of thirty-five different foods at each meal. Every food had its own separate dish, and was unseasoned, but salt was available. Each child chose different foods in different quantities, and the choice varied from day to day. As quickly as a dish was emptied it was refilled. One child took eleven helpings of lamb at one meal and nothing else. Strenuous exercise had preceded the meal, but no ill effects were noted as a result of the excessive amount of meat eaten. After one year of free choice of foods, all the children were found in much better health than when the experiment had begun. Dental decay and rickets had been reduced to a bare minimum.

Many will wonder why our diets have changed. Why we gave up the food customs established through years of trial and error. The basic reason is that mechanization has made it possible to support more people on less land; industrialization has led to the congregating of people in cities and specialization has led to a marked division between those who produce foods, and those who contribute to society in other ways. Comparatively few people now produce their own food. Production and distribution are commercialized. There is a greater variety of foods, transported over greater distances, but many of them are so processed and refined that they have lost many of the elements they contained in their natural state. Moreover, when people buy their food instead of producing it, the economic factor has a more powerful influence on the kind of diet they receive. In this situation, it is easy to lose sight of tradition and habit and because of the changes brought about in food through processing, picking green, and shipping, a diet dictated by tradition may not have the elements of former days. The great mobility of population is another factor. Coastal people moving inland tend to adopt the food habits of their neighbors and locality without any thought of their physical differences. Today in America, diets are pretty well standardized and even Europeans adopt our food customs within one or two generations after their arrival.

The greatest changes in nutrition have been from whole grain flours to white flour; from few sweets, and those natural, to refined sugar, and that in large quantities; to the use of chemical preservatives in food and the use of coffee. Those three things, white flour, sugar and coffee are the most common and most harmful elements in our diet. They have been in great use only one to two hundred years, which is a long time if you think in terms of your life and mine, but not when you think in terms of civilization as a whole. In plant life, alterations can be developed or new species brought into being, but it is a process of selection and repeated reproduction involving generations of plant life. We use scientific methods to produce plants, we are hit-and-miss about the propagation of man. To make radical dietary changes in one to two hundred years is to court disaster. The human mechanism is not adapted to such rapid changes. Our bodies are capable of adaptation, but it must be a slow process covering hundreds of generations.

The popularity of white flour is due to a very clever bit of salesmanship. Whole grain flours do not keep easily— rodents and bugs know what is good to eat. White flour keeps well and is suitable for transportation. Therefore, from the commercial point of view, white flour is a more satisfactory product. In the past, its nutritional value was not considered. Once a luxury of the rich, it soon became the desire of all people to have refined flour and sugar to grace their tables.

White flour in itself is not harmful, but by displacing more important food factors it leads to deficiencies. Vitamin B, which is so lacking in the American diet, is found in abundance in the whole grains. Now of course the baking companies fortify bread with synthetic vitamin B. But why take out the natural vitamin, only later to replace it artificially? Only a small part of what has been taken out is returned in artificially "enriched breads," and that is never as good as what is provided by mother nature. (The other vitamins—known as vitamin B complex—are lacking in our bread as well as minerals.) In the process of making white flour from whole wheat, 80% of its calcium and phosphorus is lost. It is easy to see why white flour and white flour products can be adequately described as "empty calories." White flour will put on weight, but it lacks those elements vital to nourishing a healthy body. The same applies to polished white rice and all refined grains.

Dr. Weston Price, in the 1930's, made a most notable study of the diets of primitive peoples existing in many parts of the world today. He found that where primitive people were uninfluenced by modern diet, the incidence of dental decay and other degenerative diseases was markedly low as compared with the figures tabulated among so-called civilized people. In the secluded area inhabited by primitive tribes, the diet was found to consist chiefly of whole grain, animal and sea foods, vegetables and fruits. The most desired parts of the animals were the liver, fats, heart, and kidneys. These parts by chemical analysis were found to contain more vitamins and minerals than the muscle parts, which civilized people consider particularly choice.

When white flour and sugar became part of the daily food intake for these people, dental decay, tuberculosis and other diseases flourished. Never having been exposed to these ills, no immunity to them had been established. Therefore, once their systems had become weakened through an inadequate and rapidly changing diet, they were easy victims to bacterial invasion. Even in two or three generations these people could be reduced to one-tenth their former number merely through the breakdown of their body chemical balance due to an inadequate diet.

The rate of deterioration of these hitherto immune people seems to be directly in proportion to the amount of harmful dietary intake.

Sugar and white flour were introduced to these people simultaneously in large quantities. Within one generation the effects were devastating. Among us the more gradual acceptance of these items of diet results in a less rapid, though still too rapid degeneration. Island tribes in some localities were found existing in good health upon an unvaried diet of fish, whole grains, and some wild plant life. Thus a few natural foods were found to be more productive of health than the refined, delectably concocted dishes of modern man. The percentage of dental decay among these people was negligible so long as they remained on their native diet. A recognition of the value of fish food was widespread. Even high in the Andes Mountains natives were found carrying small pouches at their waists, filled with dried fish eggs and seaweed, products which could be obtained only by making long journeys to the sea.

Among primitive people, much greater thought is given to the diet of both men and women previous to conception than is the custom in modern civilization. Long trips are made for special foods, crabs, the ashes of water hyacinths, and certain cereals, because tradition has taught that these foods have peculiar dietary values that influence the physical and mental well-being of future progeny. Dr. Price had laboratory examinations made of these special foods and found that such food customs were scientifically sound. Unusual amounts of calcium, iodine, and caroten, which affect vitamin use within the body, were found to characterize them.

Where modern diet was accepted by the natives, structural changes of the bony formation of the body were observable within one generation. Narrowed dental arches affected respiration and mastication, aiding in the onslaught of disease. Pelvic formations in women were altered and affected the bearing of children. In brief, general deterioration of the body was observed with an inevitable effect upon their mental and moral well-being.

That this process could be reversed by a return to the native diets was evidenced among the people of one of the Pacific Islands. Temporarily, the high price of copra permitted the exchange for large quantities of white flour and sugar. The children of the island rapidly developed a high rate of dental decay, although previously only a small fraction of the people had been so affected. The day came when the value of copra dropped so low that it was unprofitable for the traders to stop. The old native diet was reinstated and shortly, dental decay ceased. Dr. Price even saw open cavities where decay had stopped. Chemical balance of the body had been re-established and bacteria were no longer able to penetrate the tooth structures.

Instead of seeking economic profit through exploitation of these people, it might pay us to adopt their customs regulating health and the production of mentally and physically excellent children. By correlating the findings of all these people and using them in our own civilization, we should be able not only to equal their standards of health, but to exceed them.

Dr. Price's research proved, beyond doubt, that there is a definite relationship between nutrition and health. But unlike the natives discussed in his book, we not only want to know what things aid in establishing and maintaining health, but we want to know the chemical reason for the ability of certain foods to create certain effects. And so we have experimental laboratories trying out varied diets and food elements on animals. These experiments are valuable to the progress of nutritional understanding, but we must not forget that in as much as a rat differs from a cat in physical appearance and needs in the same degree, we differ from them both. Let us make use of all the information obtainable from animal experimentation, but let us beware of too quickly drawing conclusions as to their application to us.

There are many "unknowns" in the field of nutrition.

Laboratory experiments are constantly seeking solutions and unearthing new questions. For some years a cat experiment was carried on in California. Two groups of female cats were kept confined in wire cages. All the edible greens within reach outside the runways disappeared quickly. The diet was supposed to meet the nutritional requirements of cats as now known. It was the same for both groups of caged cats except for one thing. Half of the cats had cooked meat and half had raw meat, but evidence of malnutrition was great in both classes of cats. None of the kittens of the second generation subsisting on cooked meat lived beyond four months. The progeny of the cats eating raw meat survived through another generation. The male cats in this experiment were allowed to run free and forage for their own food. They were sleek and healthy and superior to both of the other groups. How much quicker would be the degeneration of the kittens if both parents were existing on the same diet!

Sensitivity to wheat is a common complaint among the mixed people of America, and in general it can be stated that the ancestors who determined the endocrine pattern of these people ate rye rather than wheat, which was not common in Europe, and their descendants should do likewise to avoid discomfort. Why is it that any of us tolerate wheat, since so few of our ancestors were accustomed to it? That answer undoubtedly lies in the endocrine patterns rather than in the food, yet it still constitutes a nutritional problem.

When we think of how little we knew about the subject forty years ago, or even twenty years ago, and how much has been learned in that time, it is unthinkable that we shall not continue to learn in the future.

For the present there is at least one ground upon which we are fairly safe. Our ancestors must have dined well enough for survival, or we would not be here. We also know that the more natural the diet, the fewer the degenerative diseases.

Evidence shows that our tastes and appetites can again

be depended upon to tell us what we should eat, providing we use a little intelligence as a seasoning for the food.

First of all, in order for food to be nutritive it must be wholesome. Second, and just as important to the individual, the nutritive value of food also depends upon the ability of the person to digest the food. There are some who digest fat poorly because of the lack of bile; some cannot digest meat readily due to an insufficient amount of hydrochloric acid in the stomach; while others are not able to assimilate a coarse diet, which must be digested slowly because the intestines expel the food particles enveloped in hard capsules of cellulose before the cellulose is dissolved by the bacteria of the large intestines. People who have this deficiency cannot digest whole wheat bread, cereals, and legumes very well. Everything that an individual digests with difficulty, or that goes through the intestines too fast, has little nutritive value for that person.

It is very erroneous to accept the idea that any man's needs are exactly like those of any other. There are many people and some dietitians who state that there is a specific diet that is good for everyone. What has happened is that a given individual has found that a specific diet is excellent for him, but he forgets that no other person has his specific heredity, and is thus making a mistake when he prescribes it for everyone. It may be good for other people; it most certainly will be good for those who are most like him in heredity and racial stock. We cannot accept the assembly line philosophy of diet without falling into the pitfall of food fadism.

It has been established beyond doubt that sugar, all refined foods, coffee, and alcohol are, in a fundamental sense, enemies of proper nutrition in that they are "empty calories" lacking the basic food builders required for good health. Yet, each of us has known some people who consume large amounts of these artificial foods and seem to get along relatively well. This does not mean that these hardy people are an exception to the principles of nutrition; they must have all the minerals, amino acids, and vitamins which are necessary to sustain life. It does mean that due to their particular heredity, their needs for these basic substances are probably very low. Still, in time, these people will begin to have trouble which could have been avoided had they merely followed a sound diet.

Very recently Dr. E. Cheraskin of the University of Alabama, visited one of our submarines. He noted that the officers and crew consumed on the average of 22 to 24 cups of coffee daily. Most of the men also had at least one teaspoonful of sugar in each cup. The young and vigorous can take it but it probably contributes to our V.A. Hospital population in later years.

Many diseases may be attacked nutritionally with a high degree of success if it is done with an understanding of the distinctiveness of individual needs.

It is the individual heredity of each person that endows him with his specific characteristics, and these characteristics are largely set through environment. That is why a specific diet cannot be prescribed for everyone indiscriminately. In my research with thousands of patients over the past forty years, my findings prove that certain foods are universally harmful to everyone. Those foods are as follows: Sugar and all foods made with sugar (white, brown, or raw sugar and syrups), white bread and refined grains, coffee, tea, milk (not including cream and butter), fruit and vegetable juices and hydrogenated fats. These items should never be eaten if you want your diet to be wholesome and promote good health.

One of the points about diet which seems to be difficult for most people to understand is why a person should not drink fruit juices when there is no restriction on the amount of fruit eaten.

The hunger center of the brain tells one when he has had enough food. The thirst center is for telling when one has had enough water. The throat center does not work on all liquids. When too much fruit or vegetable juices are taken the alkaline-acid balance of the body is changed. The pH of the urine is acid and should be maintained so. When the urine becomes alkaline and remains so, it is indicative of an imbalance. Calcium will precipitate in an alkaline media so that in this condition (alkaline) we may find precipitation.

The more one understands about the physiology of the body, the more one realizes how much the body knows that man's poor brain has never learned.

A specific diet cannot be prescribed as being good for everyone in that each person has a distinct heredity and has had varied experiences in his environment. This manifests itself in the functioning of the endocrine system which determines assimilation and utilization of the food we eat. A good diet is always beneficial to health, and a poor diet is always injurious to health. The degree to which a bad diet manifests itself depends upon the hereditary constitution of the person concerned. Where there is improper assimilation, it is evident that the person needs endocrine treatment specifically suited for his special needs. As a guide for a proper diet, the following lists give the foods that are wholesome and healthful, and those which should be avoided.

THE PAGE DIET FOR HEALTH

(A healthy, wholesome diet may be selected from the following list according to your special needs. A healthy diet should include foods from each area, but not necessarily each food for a given person. This list offers a wide range of recommended foods).

1. Meat, fish, sea foods, fowl, eggs, liver, and all edible organs of animals.
2. Vegetables of all kinds—raw or cooked—not overcooked.
3. Whole grain cereals or flours: oatmeal, wheat hearts, barley, millet, corn, grits, brown rice, 100% whole wheat, 100% rye. (Make sure that these are not saturated with chemical preservatives and are 100% what they are supposed to be).
4. Fresh fruits of all kinds.

5. Dried fruits (natural, no sugar added).

6. 100% whole wheat bread, 100% rye bread. (Most whole wheat and rye breads are only around 40% to 60% whole wheat or rye, the remainder is white flour).

7. Butter, heavy cream.

8. Lard (natural animal shortenings) liquid vegetable oils, i.e., corn, peanut, olive, etc. Use *no* hydrogenated shortenings.

9. Honey, pure, unpasteurized. Pure tupelo honey is the best in that it has the highest content of levulose, however, the others are good. Honey should be used in strict moderation. One can eat too much honey which can cause an upset in the balance of body chemistry.

10. Gelatin—any brand of pure, unsweetened gelatin. It is a good source of protein and may be sweetened with a little natural fruit juice. The commercial gelatins containing sugar should never be used.

11. For a beverage, which is not necessary but often pleasant, use decaffeinated coffee or *very weak* tea.

12. Natural Vitamins. Whenever vitamin supplementation is needed, natural vitamins should be used rather than synthetic ones.

13. Natural seasoning such as celery salt, bay leaves, chives, and certain combined seasonings, composed of vegetable low-sodium salts and kelp.

A CORRECTED DIET ELIMINATES THE FOLLOWING UNWHOLESOME FOODS

1. Sugar and products containing sugar. This includes white sugar, brown sugar, raw sugar, molasses, and syrups. It eliminates all sugar-containing products such as jellies, jams, preserves, cakes, pies, ice cream, sherbet, jello, gelatin desserts made with sugar, cookies, cakes, doughnuts, pastries, canned fruits, chewing gum.

2. White flour products. This includes white bread,

packaged ready cooked cereals such as cream of
wheat, cookies, cakes, noodles, macaroni, spaghetti,
and pastries.

3. Milk and milk products such as cheese. (This does
not include cream and butter which are animal fats
and are very healthful. As a substitute for milk, one
should use ⅓ cup of heavy cream to ⅔ cups of
water).

4. Hydrogenated fats. This includes margarines, solid
vegetable shortenings, peanut butter. One can find
non-hydrogenated peanut butter in most health food
stores. So many prepared foods are now made with
hydrogenated fats that it also excludes them from the
list of a healthy diet.

5. Coffee and strong tea. One may use decaffeinated
coffee. Whenever a coffee drinker stops using coffee,
it is often common for that person to have a head-
ache for one or two days; this is due to ridding the
system of the craving for caffeine; it is merely the response of the body to freeing itself from its depend-
ency upon a harmful stimulant.

6. Juices, both fruit and vegetable.

7. Synthetic vitamins, except when used along with natural vitamins in special cases.

8. Chemical preservatives. All foods preserved with
chemical preservatives. Often these preservatives are
very poisonous, and particularly after continued use,
may have very harmful effects upon the body. Read
the labels, and if the product contains chemical preservatives or food additives, avoid it. This includes
most dry breakfast cereals, most commercially produced breads, processed meats, many types of dried
fruits (for example, certain brands of raisins, certain
brands of dressings made for salads, and many other
commercially produced foods.)

9. Alcohol and alcoholic beverages. If used, use in moderation.

Vitamins

Among the many maladies which afflict mankind are the so-called "nutritional diseases" of which vitamin deficiencies are one class. These diseases can be prevented and cured merely by feeding the person enough fresh, wholesome, natural food products provided that his system can absorb them. In studying and learning about these diseases, it makes one wonder about what other diseases, even those that are caused by bacteria, may have their origin in an improper diet and inefficient nutrition. It is well known that a healthy body, though exposed to infectious diseases, is not likely to contract them. Disease germs can grow only in an unhealthy body. The process may be likened to a chain. When one link is broken, the strength of the whole chain is broken. A diet which results in a vitamin deficiency may be the link which breaks and thus brings on a nutritional disease which, if not corrected, will be fatal.

Hippocrates described scurvy in ancient times, and the disease seemed to especially plague armies in the field and cities that underwent siege for long periods of time. Later, following the discovery of America, when long sea voyages became common, scurvy became common among sailors. Little was known about what caused scurvy and less about its cure, though elaborate theories and remedies were prescribed—most of them worthless, and none completely effective.

In 1553 Cartier made his second voyage to Newfoundland. Of his 103-man crew 100 developed agonizing scurvy and were in great anguish when the Iroquois Indians of Quebec came to their rescue with what was described as a "miraculous cure." The Iroquois Indians gave the sick sailors an infusion of bark and leaves of the pine tree. In 1553 Admiral Sir Richard Hawkins noted that during his career upon the high seas 10,000 seamen under his command had died of scurvy. He further recorded that in his experience sour oranges and lemons had been most effective in curing the disease. Yet these observations had no sweeping effect in bringing about an awareness of what could prevent scurvy, and the observations of this admiral went unheeded.

James Lind, a British naval surgeon, who later became the chief physician of the Naval Hospital at Portsmouth, England, published in 1753 a book stating explicitly how scurvy could be eliminated simply by supplying sailors with lemon juice. He cited many case histories from his experience as a naval surgeon at sea; he proved that such things as mustard cress, tamarinds, oranges and lemons would prevent scurvy. In fact, anything which contains enough vitamin C, which is most abundant in citrus fruit, tomatoes, and to a lesser degree in most green vegetables and other fruits, will prevent scurvy.

You might rightfully expect that Dr. Lind would have been highly honored and praised for his great contribution. The reverse was true. He was ridiculed and became frustrated. He remarked bitterly: "Some persons cannot be brought to believe that a disease so fatal and so dreadful can be cured or prevented by such easy means." They would have more faith in an elaborate composition dignified with the title of "an antiscorbutic golden elixir" or the like. The "some persons" to whom Dr. Lind referred were My Lords of the Admiralty and the other physicians. In fact, they ignored Dr. Lind's advice for forty years. One sea captain did take his advice—the now famous Captain James Cook, who stocked his ships with an ample supply of fresh fruits. The Royal Society honored Captain Cook in 1776 for his success, but the officials of the navy ignored the report. It was not until 1794, the year of Dr. Lind's death, that the first British navy squadron was supplied with lemon juice for a voyage of twenty-three weeks. On that voyage there was not one case of scurvy, yet another decade was to pass before regulations were enacted requiring the sailors to drink a daily ration of lemon juice to prevent scurvy. With this enactment, scurvy disappeared from the British Navy, and after the lapse of another sixty years, the same regulation was applied to the merchant marine fleet. A century after Captain Cook's great success in preventing scurvy on his ship, LeRoy de Mericourt praised Captain Cook's therapy before the French Academy of Medicine, but his words were received with great doubt and hostility. One would think with the publication by Dr. Lind in 1753 that the world would readily heed his work, but it was almost a century later before the wisdom of his teaching became well known and even later before it became general practice in the prevention of scurvy. It takes a long time for something new to become accepted. Louis Pasteur had the same difficulty in getting his discoveries accepted—that harmful bacteria cause infectious diseases—and it was only in his later life, following ridicule, that his great contributions to mankind were recognized. Likewise, the body chemistry approach to preventing degenerative disease is only gradually coming to be accepted and recognized—the day when it will be generally recognized is still in the future.

Scurvy was the first vitamin deficiency disease to be treated successfully before its exact cause was discovered, but there were others. The other major ones were beriberi and pellagra.

During the latter part of the last century beriberi became a prevalent disease in the Far East, especially in Indonesia. A Dutch doctor, Christian Eijkman, (1858-1930), was sent from Holland to investigate the ravages of beriberi. He felt certain that it was caused by a germ and he was determined to find the germ causing the disease. People suffering from beriberi develop nervous and paralytic symptoms and finally die an agonizing death. It was only by chance that Eijkman finally found out what caused beriberi. In his experiments he was feeding chickens polished rice—rice left on the plates of patients—in an effort to find the germ that caused the disease and they developed the disease. A new superintendent ordered this stopped as white rice was considered a superior food not to be wasted on chickens. Following this the chickens, which had developed beriberi on the white rice, were fed brown or unpolished rice. To his amazement, the chickens fully recovered. He followed up this observation by checking prisoners who were fed the cheaper brown rice and only one case of beriberi was found. In another prison where polished rice was given the prisoners, only one had escaped beriberi. It was difficult for Eijkman to give up the germ theory for beriberi, and he did so only in 1906, but his observations proved that there was something in the brown covering of rice which prevented beriberi. Polished rice, or white rice as we call it today, had lost this something, and people whose diet was largely composed of white rice were the ones who developed beriberi. Yet, Eijkman's discovery was not accepted at once—it took a long time. It was found that the "something" in brown rice which prevented beriberi was vitamin B. The word vitamin was coined by the Polish scientist, Casimir Funk, who was the first man to successfully isolate and extract the chemical factor in the rice polishings which prevent beriberi.

In 1906, Sir Federick Gowland Hopkins, as a result of his significant research into food, stated that: "No animal can live upon a mixture of pure protein, fat and carbohydrate, and even when the necessary inorganic material is carefully supplied, the animal still cannot flourish." His work opened up new horizons with regard to health but did not make a great impact as the fact and theory of bacterial disease was in vogue. Today, after great success in conquering diseases of bacterial origin, that influence and emphasis is still overwhelmingly dominant within the field of the medical arts. But little by little, as one can see, the way is being paved for emphasis upon the major realm of prevention—prevention of degenerative diseases which have their origin in heredity and particularly in the diet and nutrition of modern man.

Europe and the United States have not had to face the problem of beriberi, but they have been plagued with pellagra—a kindred disease to beriberi. Pellagra is characterized by dermatitis of the skin areas which are exposed to the air constantly—the hands, face, legs, and neck. Digestive troubles develop and are accompanied by dizziness. Eventually mental disturbances manifest themselves and are followed by insanity and death, often by suicide. At first it was definitely thought that the disease was caused by germs, that it was infectious in origin. Joseph Goldberger finally succeeded in proving that the disease was due exclusively to eating habits. It was prevalent in the deep South where the poorer people, who could not afford fresh meat and dairy products and did not choose, due to customs, to eat green vegetables, were the ones who primarily suffered from pellagra. They lived mainly on corn bread, salt pork and syrup. Of course, corn bread is a healthful food but life cannot be sustained on it alone. Salt pork loses much of its vitality in being cured, while syrup is merely liquid sugar. The diet did not supply something which was necessary for healthy living and whatever it lacked produced the deficiency disease of pellagra. It was found that if these people were fed large quantities of yeast, eggs and a well-rounded diet, they recovered rapidly. Pellagra only affects those whose diets are extremely limited to foods lacking qualities which make for sound health. In 1937 it was discovered that the element lacking from the diet of pellagra sufferers was nicotinic acid, often called PP—pellagra preventive—which is one of the B vitamins. Later a whole complex of B vitamins was found; this complexity is amply illustrated by the momentous discovery in recent years of vitamin B_{12}.

The discovery and isolation of vitamins falls within the Twentieth Century—in fact, new ones are still being discovered and some that have been discovered are little understood. The background leading to the discoveries was slow and tedious. It was due to the tenacity of purpose of a few conscientious scientists with the element of luck playing its hand. We shall turn to the individual vitamins now and see what their importance is to health and what the result of their absence can produce. Scurvy and pellagra are examples of the complete absence of two vitamins, but there can be lesser deficiencies which will manifest themselves in the health of the individual in direct ratio to the deficiency and requirements of his body.

Vitamin C, also known as ascorbic acid, is abundant in nature; it is found in large quantities in citrus fruits, tomatoes, green peppers, green leafy vegetables, fruits, Irish potatoes, radishes, liver and fresh meat. It is vitamin C which is necessary to prevent scurvy. Prolonged deficiencies of vitamin C may lead to anemia, defective teeth, and local hemorrhages of the gums and membranes of the nose and mouth. Vitamin C, in some way not fully understood, influences the workings of the endocrine glands. People deprived of vitamin C are exceptionally prone to general infection. Whenever the body is fighting an invasion of parasites, vitamin C is used at a rapid rate. Surveys have shown this to be true of patients suffering from tuberculosis, acute arthritis and osteomyelitis, and it seems that a deficiency of vitamin C renders one more susceptible to the common cold as well as infectious diseases in general. It has been found that the white blood cells, which are the body's chief fighters against invading germs, are richly endowed with vitamin C.

The human body cannot store or manufacture its own vitamin C as can most other animals; therefore it must be taken into the body each day. It has been estimated that at least 53 per cent of the population of the U.S. suffers from vitamin C deficiency to some degree. Smoking and the inhaling of cigarette smoke burns up vitamin C at a fast rate; it has been stated that the smoking and inhaling of one cigarette uses up 25 milligrams of vitamin C; therefore smokers would be well advised to supplement their diet with vitamin C. It is easy to determine if one has enough vitamin C; when there is an ample supply within the body it will be present in the urine; its absence in the urine shows that there is a deficiency. Vitamin C is necessary for healthy teeth, bones, gums, blood vessels, intercellular substances, and as a guard against infectious diseases.

Closely related to vitamin C is a substance found in the pulp (not the juice) of citrus fruit, red peppers, tea, and other foods containing vitamin C; this substance has been termed vitamin P. It seems that vitamin P aids the body in retaining vitamin C and strengthens the capillary walls.

The modern name for what was once called vitamin B is now vitamin B complex. It is now known that there are at least twelve different classifications, or factors, of vitamin B—all inter-related but distinct. All of these are present in the same sources of food and are primarily found in the outer covering of rice (brown rice)—non-polished rice), the outer layer of wheat, the outer layer of oats, millet, rye and other grains, beans and seeds, the germ of grains, the yolk of eggs and in leafy vegetables. Modern civilization, with its dependence upon refined grains, has robbed itself of its major source of the B complex vitamins. Beriberi, which was due to living mainly on polished rice, developed because the body was deprived of the vital vitamin B complex, present in the outer covering of rice. It may be described as an aristocratic disease in origin. At first only the royalty and nobility—the wealthy—could afford polished rice. Eventually everyone wanted to eat it; and since the king and wealthy preferred it, white rice was considered to be vastly superior to the unpolished brown rice. So the people began to eat refined rice rather than using it in its natural state. The results were disastrous—beriberi which resulted in agonizing death. As a parallel development, our dependence on refined grains, mainly white flour, is the same. We are robbing ourselves of the vital natural minerals and vitamins which are found in the germ of the grain and the outer coverings; that is why whole wheat, whole rye, and other whole grains are superior to refined grains. They give us nothing but pure carbohydrate—something that does not exist in a natural state.

A deficiency of vitamin B_1 (thiamin) interrupts or even stops the assimilation of sugars, while the poisonous residual products cause unhealthy reactions in the nervous system. It is possible that the loss of appetite characteristic of vitamin B_1 deficiency, may be due to the building up in the blood stream of starches and sugars insufficiently broken down. The general characteristics of vitamin B₁ deficiency are nervousness, loss of appetite, loss of muscle tone, digestive upsets, vague aches and pains, constipation and mental depression. Vitamin B₁ is necessary for proper digestion, a healthy nervous system, and aids the heart and muscles in functioning properly.

The anti-beriberi vitamin was called "B" but later research discovered that it is a complex vitamin composed mainly of an antineuritic factor termed B₁ along with a factor necessary for metabolism called "B₂" also known as lactoflavin or riboflavin, which influences growth by controlling absorption of food by the small intestines. In this respect, a good diet is necessary to promote the bodily aspects of good nutrition. Absence of B₁ and B₂ from the diet causes pellagra, the result of which is insanity and agonizing death if it is not treated; the treatment is simple and easy, yet many people in the U.S. still become afflicted with this disease each year. A prolonged deficiency of vitamin B₂ may lead to dryness of the hair and skin, skin trouble, reddening of the lips, inflammation of the mouth with sores in and about the mouth. Vitamin B₂ promotes healthy skin, mouth and eyes, and an exchange of oxygen in the body cells.

Vitamin B₆, also known as pyridoxine, is related to protein and fat metabolism and is necessary for healthy nerves, skin, and muscles. Its absence from the diet may lead to skin eruptions, pronounced nervous disorders, inability to sleep and general irritability. Vitamin B₁₂, one of the newest discoveries of the B complex vitamins, is necessary for blood-building, prevention of anemia, a good appetite and for normal growth in children.

There is a whole series of the other B complex vitamins as follows: pantothenic acid, folic acid, choline, inositol, biotin or vitamin H, niacin, and para-amino-benzoic acid. The role of these vitamins is not fully understood at the present, but it is known that they are necessary for healthy functioning of the digestive system, liver, intestinal tract, and for good blood-building. A prolonged deficiency of these vitamins of the B complex family usually results in abnormal growth, specific types of anemia, and perhaps other unfortunate consequences not yet fully explored.

One of the oldest diseases recorded in history is night blindness. In ancient times it was treated by feeding the patient liver. Hippocrates, the father of medicine, prescribed as a remedy for night blindness, ox liver dipped in honey. Around the middle of the nineteenth century authorities began to suspect that night blindness was dietary in origin. Not until the twentieth century was it discovered that the disease was due to a dietary deficiency. A group of experimental animals were fed on a casein-dextrin-lactose diet with the result that they developed night blindness. When butter and egg yolks were added to their diet, they recovered rapidly. Having proved that the ailment was alimentary, the discoverers named the element necessary for its prevention vitamin A.

It is generally characteristic of the vitamins that each one performs a number of functions. If the condition of night blindness is not treated successfully, it will degenerate into a condition known as exerophthalmia, in which the cornea dries up and becomes ulcerated and inflamed. In fact, night blindness is the first warning of vitamin A deficiency and of more serious trouble to develop if the condition is not remedied. Vitamin A deficiency will lead to unhealthy developments in the mucous membranes of the respiratory, alimentary and genito-urinary organs in addition to the eyes and tear glands. A healthy mucous membrane is able to resist infection and oppose bacterial attack while a vitamin A deficiency, which weakens the mucous membranes, breaks down such resistance. It is possible that vitamin A deficiency may play a role in one's susceptibility to colds and sore throat.

Butter, eggs, carrots, string beans, cucumbers, tomatoes, paprika, and liver are rich in vitamin A. In northern climates, during winter months, due to a lack of food rich in vitamin A, the body may become deficient in this substance. Even butter during the winter months is deficient in vitamin A as the cows have been fed on dry feeds rather than pastured on fresh, green grass and clover. Vitamin A is especially present in very large quantities in the livers of fish, particularly such fish as cod and halibut which is the source of commercial vitamin A.

Rickets, which especially attacks children, is due to a vitamin D deficiency. Fortunately, the body can manufacture its own vitamin D or obtain it from foods rich in it. The body requires only very minute amounts of vitamin D, yet many people do not even get this tiny amount. The skin contains a compound called ergosterol, which when exposed to ultra-violet rays of the sun is converted to vitamin D. As simple as it may seem, many people in the United States do not get enough vitamin D, especially in the winter months when most of their time is spent inside. The ultra-violet rays of the sun will not go through glass, hence inside, sunlight is of no value in this respect. Vitamin D is necessary for normal calcium and phosphorus metabolism which makes for strong and healthy bones, and its absence results not only in rickets, but spasmophilia, osteomalacia, and other diseases which are manifestations of abnormal calcium and phosphorus balance.

Vitamin D is found in largest quantities of cod liver oil, and during the winter months it would be wise for children, as well as adults, to take a small spoonful each day. It is also found in mackerel, herring, sprats, egg yolks, butter, and animal livers.

Man no doubt never suffered from a deficiency of vitamin D until he became so highly civilized that large numbers of people spend the greater part of their lives inside buildings, and when not in buildings in automobiles. A normal, healthy body given a chance by being properly exposed to the sun will manufacture its own vitamin D. Of course, if the body chemistry is not functioning normally, the mechanism of the body for making and absorbing vitamin D may be impaired. It is fortunate that man can, through proper nutrition, get enough vitamin D through a good, natural diet.

Vitamin D is one of those vitamins in which a word of caution must be given. Too much can be very harmful to the body. So can overexposure to the sun. It is like good fertilizer—a plant needs a certain amount and will die without it, but with too much it will also die—just enough and no more must be present for good health. Too much vitamin D can result in intense headaches, nausea, vomiting, profuse perspiration, loss of appetite, loss of energy, and weariness. One does not have to worry about manufacturing too much from the sunlight, but caution must be exercised in taking it orally in the form of cod liver oil or in pill form.

Vitamin D is necessary to insure healthy bones and teeth and to aid in regulating calcium and phosphorus metabolism. Vitamin D deficiency may result in poor bone and tooth development in children, muscle weakness, tooth degeneration, bone disorders, and a number of specific diseases previously listed.

It was long believed that nutrition could not affect the reproductive cells of the body, but it was demonstrated around 1925 that rats fed on white refined flour became sterile. Subsequent research proved that the cause was due to an anti-sterility factor found in wheat germ which has been given the name vitamin E. Vitamin E plays a part in regulating sexual development, and much sterility is due to its absence from the diet. Besides a factor in sterility, failure of pregnancy to take place and miscarriage, it has something to do with muscular and nervous diseases. Recent research also indicates that vitamin E has an influence on the pituitary and thyroid glands of the body and some authorities maintain that it is of great importance in the prevention and cure of heart and blood vessel disturbances. The major source of vitamin E is whole wheat (the wheat germ), brown rice, 100 per cent rye, corn and whole grain cereals such as oatmeal and grits; it is also found in lesser quantities in fresh beef, liver, eggs, fresh vegetables and vegetables oils. In that so little whole wheat bread is eaten today, many people no doubt do not get the minimum amount of vitamin E. Many of the cereals, such as cream of wheat, are made from refined grains and are thus lacking in this vital element. In switching from whole grain breads to refined white breads, man has unwittingly robbed himself of the most important factors that those foods contain in their natural state. Even most 100 per cent whole wheat breads which are available in the markets, are not desirable in that they have had a chemical preservative added which is a foreign element for the body and hence, probably harmful. Whole wheat bread does not keep as well as white bread so a larger amount of chemical preservative is needed.

Another known vitamin is K. It has something to do with the formation of prothrombin, without which, blood will not coagulate. The vitamin is therefore known as the anti-hemorrhage factor or the blood clotting vitamin. This is very important because when the body is injured by a cut or internal injury causing bleeding within the body, the victim will bleed to death if the blood does not clot. Vitamin K is found in large quantities in most green vegetables, tomatoes and pork liver. Withering or yellowing of vegetables appears to have no effect on vitamin K.

Vitamins are necessary for a healthy body and mind, but too many of them can be harmful. This is particularly true of the fat soluble vitamins—A, D, E and K. An overdose of vitamin A is believed to affect the liver while it has already been stated what too much vitamin D can do. There seems to be no danger with the water soluble vitamins—vitamins B, C, etc. Many of the vitamins complement the work of others: for example, vitamin D opposes the actions of vitamin A and E, while vitamin A and D reinforce actions of vitamin B. This shows the danger of overdosage of synthetic or drugstore vitamins. In natural foods, vitamins exist in proper proportions. When vitamin supplements are taken, and in this modern world when we eat mainly processed and refined foods, it is often wise to use them, but only natural vitamins should be used. Synthetic vitamins are the pure substance without the pressure of other vitamins and enzymes which must be present for the body to utilize them properly. It is something like oxygen; the body must have oxygen to live, but pure oxygen breathed into the lungs will do great damage—the lungs are equipped to handle oxygen as it is in the atmosphere, not in the pure, rarefied form. The same is true of vitamins for human use.

It is difficult to say exactly how much of a certain vitamin or vitamins a person needs. This is due to the individual heredity. On the basis of what has been learned with reference to the relationship between heredity and biochemical processes of the body, it seems that each individual has a pattern of needs that is quantitatively different from that of others. The numerous chemical processes that take place within our bodies do so with unequal efficiencies as is regulated by our body chemistry. For that reason our needs for the various vitamins, minerals, and food stuffs are quantitatively unequal. In other words, it depends on the constitution of the individual which is determined by heredity and what he has done to his body over the years.

Some vitamins do not keep very well. The destruction of vitamins is due to their oxidation, which in turn depends upon heat and the presence of oxygen and the acid-alkaline balance of the medium in which the vitamins are found or placed. Vitamin C is especially sensitive to heat. Cooking destroys it in most vegetables and fruits with the exception of the Irish potato where cooking increases the concentration of vitamin C. However, in the absence of air, vitamin C can be heated to a very high temperature without damage. It is much less susceptible to deterioration in an acid medium than in an alkali. The loss of vitamin content in preserved foods is caused by their sensitivity to heat. Heating foods above the boiling point in the presence of air destroys vitamin C and partially destroys A and B_1. For that reason vegetables should never be overcooked. Artificial drying by heat also affects vitamins in the same way. Vitamins A and B_1 are little destroyed by cooking while D, E, and B_2 show no change whatsoever. Curing meat by smoking causes a loss of vitamin content. Cold temperatures, while slowing chemical and biological processes, cause little or no change in vitamins. Fresh foods are always richer in vitamin content than canned foods, processed foods, preserved foods and cured foods; this is particularly true of vitamin C. It is wise to eat as much of one's food in the form of fresh meat, whole grains and fresh vegetables as is possible.

The question may well arise, "How did we ever get along before we knew there were such things as vitamins?" The answer is that they are so widespread in nature that as long as we were living on natural foods and living in a natural manner, our needs in vitamins were automatically supplied.

We must remember that there is no necessity to rush to the drugstore to purchase these all-important vitamins. They are in our foods. All we have to do is refrain from taking them out. The chief means by which they are lost is through refining certain foods which might better be called devitalizing foods.

It is always best to get your vitamins the natural way through wholesome foods.

The most important and least publicized thing about vitamins is their chemical formula. Most vitamins are made of varying proportions of carbon, hydrogen, and oxygen, elements so essential to growth that no plant can exist without them, elements so common that they can be found anywhere in air, water and sunshine. A few vitamins do have nitrogen, phosphorus, and sulphur but these minerals are quite plentiful and are still common to our soils. So in the last analysis, our food contains plenty of vitamins if grown on good soil and if we do not destroy them in the process of preparation. Our bodies are capable of assimilating the necessary quantity of these vitamins from our food just so long as we are chemically in balance—when we have good body chemistry.

Minerals

In addition to fats, proteins, carbohydrates and vitamins, minerals are also necessary to sustain life. The most important carrier of minerals, water, seems so obvious that we take it for granted. The average body contains around fifty quarts of water and expels about four quarts each day through the urine, feces, perspiration and respiration. Man drinks only a part of this water because the foods he eats are largely made up of water. For example, vegetables are 90 per cent or more water, potatoes 80 per cent, meat and eggs some 70 per cent, and even bread, which has been baked and lost a great quantity of its water, contains from 35 to 40 per cent water. Water is so necessary to life that death results if one is deprived of it for a short period of time.

Most people prefer soft water to hard water because soap does not lather readily in the latter. However, hard water is much better for the body and may prolong life according to Dr. Henry A. Schroeder as reported in the April, 1960 edition of the Medical Journal. In the states where the water is hard, Dr. Schroeder found that there was a low death rate from heart and artery diseases. It has not been determined exactly what the agent in hard water is which helps prevent heart and artery diseases, but it may be that alkaline water gives greater protection to arteries. Acid waters which cause and build up rust in pipes may also act in such a way that they pick up impurities and cause deposits in the arteries—the body's pipes. Many people add softeners to their water, but for the water used for drinking and cooking, it would be wiser to use hard water.

The fluids of the body are not pure water, but actually a salt solution. The body is constantly excreting salt solutions with the urine, excrement, perspiration and tears, so man must eat relatively large quantities of salt to replenish the loss. Due to excessive perspiration in summer, many people need more salt than they do in the winter. The molecules of salt contained in solution form electrically charged particles called ions. The charges that these ions receive make them especially reactive chemically; since they form a current while they are moving through a solution, they confer electrical conductivity upon the solutions in which they are suspended. Thus these ions are very important in the body processes of the organism. Many people worry about their intake of salt and even go on a salt-free diet. However, it has been my experience that when one has balanced body chemistry, he need not worry about the amount of salt which he eats. Salt is necessary for a healthy body. In a healthy person, appetite will dictate one's need for salt. In treating people of various symptoms by taking them off salt, temporary relief may be rendered. However, the basic problem of establishing sound body chemistry is not approached, with the result that the patient rarely regains sound health.

Much is known today of the vitamin requirements of the body but little publicity has been given to our mineral needs. We all know that calcium and phosphorus are necessary requirements of the body, but there are also numerous other mineral elements which are essential if the body is to be maintained in a state of good health. Some of them, including sodium, potassium, and magnesium, occur in fairly large quantities. Our food fortunately contains large amounts of these minerals and nutritionists are of the belief that no deficiencies are likely to exist in the diet of the population of the United States in this respect.

There are many other minerals, however, which are essential to adequate nutrition which have an importance much greater than their bulk would indicate. Some of them are needed in very minute amounts, so minute that they are designated as "trace minerals." Seaweed is an excellent source of these as considerable amounts of land minerals have been washed into the sea by rain. The Japanese recognize the value of sea plants, which are as varied as those of the land, and use as many as twenty different kinds in their diet. Many primitive people, as well, are versed in the value of these sea growths.

Only about a dozen of the trace minerals are known to be essential, but it is suspected by many nutritionists that eventually all the minerals ordinarily found in the earth's crust will be found to play some part in the mechanism of the body. According to Alfred Shohl, M.D., "the functions of minerals are so important that they may well be said to control life itself." They feed the endocrines and aid in controlling the pressures of the intricate water system of our bodies.

In the *Yearbook Of Agriculture,* 1939 the United States Department of Agriculture treats the nutrition of plants, animals, and men in one volume This is as it should be, for the fundamentals of nutrition are the same, be it plants, animals or men. All living matter has developed as environment directed. Each succeeding generation of each living organism has had members poorly fitted to meet the environment. Some were not so well fitted to survive as others, and the well fitted were better able to transmit their ability to succeeding generations. Each region of the earth has different environmental conditions, therefore, the organisms of different regions have different qualities, each having that set of qualities best suited for survival in its regions. The result has been the survival of the fittest.

The first great distinction in the nutritional requirement of living matter is in the use of inorganic elements by plant life and the use of organic material in animal life. Even in this respect there is no sharp line of demarcation. Certain plants, like the fly-catcher, have the ability to use certain organic materials, and animals can use certain inorganic materials such as common salt or sodium chloride, and even to a certain degree the salts of other minerals. In general, however, the chief distinction between animal and plant life is the ability of the plant to use the inorganic and the inability of the animal to do so.

Climate and soil conditions differ in various parts of the world and eventually through the law of survival of the fittest, one plant developed to meet a certain set of environmental conditions, while another developed to meet another. Eventually these characteristics became so fixed that any great change in environment proved disastrous. Certain varieties of the cactus plant became adapted to the desert and under conditions suitable for most plants, they do not thrive so well. Certain trees will grow in warm climates, but will perish in colder climates and vice versa.

Even among plants of the same species, great differences in desirable environmental conditions occur. For example, corn adapted to Mexico does not do so well in Minnesota.

Likewise the same rules of development apply to animal life. One type requires plant material exclusively, another type requires a mixed diet, still another lives on products of the land and another on products of the sea. Many thousands of generations are required to produce changes to meet new environmental conditions. Fortunately, in nature, climate and other environmental conditions change rather slowly so that the step over one or a few generations is slight. If it were otherwise, the ability of the organism to change would be outpaced. But even the slow changes of nature have been too rapid. We find today evidences of organisms extinct through their inability to change fast enough.

We tend to lose sight of the fact that man is also an animal, a living organism. We like to think that we are different. We still have animal bodies which are just as subject to the laws of nature as the bodies of dogs, birds and cattle. Men as well as animals have to adapt themselves to the conditions of the regions in which they live. Some of these regions have conditions more favorable for development than others, and as a result, size and height of people vary.

Centuries ago the Shetland Islands were uninhabited by horses of any kind until some were cast ashore from a wrecked vessel. The horses multiplied and soon vegetation became insufficient for their needs. They learned to eat seaweed which was cast upon the shores in great quantities. Seaweed is a very excellent food but it contains only a small amount of calcium. Calcium became the limiting factor in the growth of succeeding generations of horses, until this compromise with nature became fixed. Today Shetland horses are called Shetland ponies because of their miniature size. Even after several generations of eating the same food as full sized horses, their size does not seem to be much greater. Their characteristics have become more or less fixed. A new variation has been developed.

A similar process of evolution has affected man. Japanese, like the ponies of the Shetland Islands have had to subsist upon calcium deficient foods and their stature is a reflection of this condition. It would seem that this limitation as to size is not very well fixed in the Japanese for the second and third generations living in the United States show an increased average height over that of their ancestors and that of the people still in Japan.

To a less noticeable extent, other peoples show their adaptation to different environmental conditions. These different environmental conditions are not always readily evident. They depend on variation of the food grown in the different habitats. Such is the case with the three main divisions of the white race; the Nordic, the Alpine and the Mediterranean.

The sea is the soil of the foods grown in the sea, just as the ground is the soil of land-grown foods. But whereas the soil of the sea is relatively constant in quantity of minerals, the soil of the land varies to a great extent. As a result, sea food has a stable content of the minerals, while foods grown upon land have a different and varying content.

Not only do land soils differ in their origin which would make for different mineral content, but they also differ in their age and exposure to the leaching effects of rainfall. It is well known that in the mountainous regions and in certain other sections of the earth, an almost total deficiency of iodine exists. This is chiefly because the salts of iodine are relatively soluble and through the centuries have been washed into the sea. Certain peoples of the earth have learned to get along with a minimum of these soluble minerals. Curiously enough, these inland-living people usually have round heads, while the coastal people generally have long heads. Wherever there is iodine in the soil there will be iodine in the rivers running from that region. The plants growing in the soil will have their content of iodine and the people and animals eating the plants will have their share. It is a strange commentary on the reasoning of some of our health officials that to supply an iodine deficiency they would put iodine in the drinking water; in the outlet instead of the inlet so-to-speak, and where plants which might change the inorganic iodine to the organic have no chance to do so. If the state would instead require an iodine content in fertilizers, the people would be far more effectively served. An even more direct and inexpensive method would be the eating of iodine-containing foods such as seaweed as do the Japanese and many other peoples of the earth. In fact, all sea foods are rich in not only iodine but in numerous minerals and particularly trace minerals. We should eat more sea foods—fish, crabs, lobsters, oysters, clams, and shrimp.

Minerals and vitamins are well understood to be essential in nutrition, but there is no exact knowledge as to all the functions they perform. However, there is evidence that they are necessary to glandular function. Perhaps they are necessary as constituents of glandular secretions, or perhaps as catalysts essential to the manufacture of these secretions by the glands. But what is more probable is that they act in both capacities. Iodine for instance is known to be an ingredient of thyroxin, the secretion of the thyroid, and zinc is essential in the manufacture of insulin; so here we have examples of an ingredient and a catalyst.

A further indication of the use of vitamins and trace minerals by the glandular organs is that analysis shows these organs are plentifully supplied by both, while the rest of the body is found to contain very little. When trace minerals are deficient in the foods of those people who especially need them, the effect is apparently on the endocrines, for the body chemistry is altered.

One of the most important functions of the trace minerals is their influence upon calcium and phosphorus metabolism. Without them, the endocrines and the autonomic system lose balance and with this goes loss of calcium-phosphorus balance. By replacing needed trace minerals in the diet it is possible, in many instances, to balance the assimilation of calcium and phosphorus. This effect is not immediate for it is not direct. The endocrines must first respond to the needed trace minerals. Sometimes this is rather quickly done and sometimes slowly. The amount of time depends upon the ability of the endocrines to respond. The old idea that vitamin D was solely concerned in the assimilation of calcium and phosphorus must be discarded. Vitamin D is no more important than many other factors. Anything that influences body chemistry influences calcium-phosphorus levels, and all of the essentials of nutrition—proteins, carbohydrates, fats, water, vitamins and minerals as well as some of the nonessentials such as sugar and other drugs—play their part in this regard.

In *Food and Life,* a publication of the United States Department of Agriculture, it is stated that many American diets do not provide near enough of the essential minerals and vitamins necessary for sound health. Minerals are largely disregarded, but they are just as essential to good health as are the other necessary ingredients.

The mineral elements required for the building of the body fall into two categories—plastic and catalytic. The plastic minerals undergo metabolic change in the body; these minerals include calcium, phosphorus, sulphur, potassium, and chlorine; these minerals are those of construction and regulate the alkalinity of the body fluids. The catalytic minerals—those which cause changes in other elements to take place without themselves changing—comprise iron, zinc, copper, manganese, and iodine. They are required for the manufacture of such vital life substances as thyroxine and hemoglobin. Cellulose is also needed although it, like water, undergoes practically no change and is eliminated. Both cellulose and water are necessary for dilution and solution and play an important role in the assimilation of food and the general functions of the body.

The human body contains approximately three pounds of calcium found largely in the bones where it is deposited. Calcium is necessary for healthy bones, teeth, nerves and muscles. Calcium also has a sedative effect upon the cells, nerves and brain, in that it contracts the ultramicroscopic pores in the cell walls. That is why it is often prescribed for relaxing the muscles. Calcium metabolism or the ability of the body to absorb calcium, is controlled by vitamins and hormones.

Vitamin D for example, fixes calcium and phosphorus in the bone structures. Milk has long been considered the best source of calcium, but H. D. Sherman reports that calcium deficiency is one of the most common dietary deficiencies in the United States. Yet milk consumption in the United States is the highest in the world. The answer, of course, lies in the part played by vitamins and hormones. When these are not present nor functioning correctly, calcium will not be absorbed properly no matter how much is put into the digestive tract; however, it may have adverse effects in causing a tendency for kidney stones to form. Actually, when body chemistry is functioning properly and when the body is supplied with a good, natural diet, the body can take the calcium out of the food which is eaten and there is no need to drink milk.

Different soils over the world vary greatly in calcium content, but even in those soils where the soil is deficient in calcium, the population shows no calcium deficiency, and it should be stressed that these people do not drink milk. Most all vegetables and foods contain some calcium. In getting enough calcium for the body, the major problem is not how much calcium is eaten, but the ability of the body to absorb it from the food eaten.

The human body contains almost 3 pounds of calcium and approximately 2 pounds of phosphorus. Calcium and phosphorus unite in the body to form calcium phosphate. Although phosphorus is extremely poisonous in its pure form, it is not toxic when combined with other elements as is done by the human body to form essentials for health. It is phosphorus, in combination with calcium, that is essential for the formation of sound, healthy teeth and bones which are made up primarily of calcium phosphate. Meat, beans, peas, and potatoes are rich in phosphorus, but the best source of phosphorus for humans is meat and eggs—animal protein—since it is most similar to that of the human body and is readily assimilated without having to undergo reconstruction. Phosphorus is also contained in the complex fat and protein compounds which are necessary for the vital bodily processes since they are present in the essential cell structures, in the cell nucleus, in the nerve cells, and even in the sex cells. The most thoroughly known phosphorus fat is lecithin. Both calcium and phosphorus are found within the blood. It is calcium and phosphorus that provide a clear index to the efficiency of body chemistry. Years ago I discovered that the proper ratio of calcium to phosphorus in the blood was 2½ milligrams of calcium to 1 milligram of prosphorus per 100 cc of blood. One of the most important factors in establishing sound body chemistry is in getting a 2½ to 1 ratio of calcium-phosphorus in the blood. This is accomplished by administering the hormone supplement, in minute dosage, to the individual according to his specific needs and through a sound, wholesome diet. As has been noted, calcium and phosphorus metabolism in the body is governed by the endocrine glands. Assimilation of calcium and phosphorus is mainly dependent upon glandular action, rather than the eating of large amounts of food containing these elements. Phosphorus, in an organic form usable by the body, is necessary for healthy bones and teeth and for the utilization of calcium and vitamin D.

The average sulphur content of the body is 100 grams. Each cell has a trace of sulphur but most of it is concentrated in the brain, the finger and toe nails, and the hair. Red hair has the highest content of sulphur. A sulphur deficiency results in brittle finger and toe nails and brittle hair. Sulphur is found in high quantities in oatmeal, eggs, beans, lentils, onions, radishes, garlic and other vegetables. The exact function of sulphur in the human metabolism is not known, but is essential for a healthy body. Sulphur plays some part in a number of vital processes. For example, where certain sulphur containing amino acids, such as cystin are present, they give off carbonic acid which is immediately transformed into taurin which goes into the liver. There it combines with other substances and passes into the intestines along with the bile. Sulphur unites with potassium cyanide to form a substance which is believed to play an important part in the body's defensive mechanism in protecting itself against poisonous cyanides.

Little is known of the part potassium plays in the human body, but certainly it must be important as small quantities of it are present in all parts of the body, particularly within the cells. Osmotic balance between the contents of the cells and their surrounding fluids depends greatly upon potassium. When meat is being cooked, a considerable portion of the potassium content passes into the broth. When this is eaten in the form of a soup, bouillon, or consomme, it results in a stimulatory effect upon the digestive organism. This is given as one good reason for beginning a meal with a meat broth soup.

It seems that manganese, in minute amounts, is essential for human existence; however, its particular function within the body is not fully understood. The greatest amounts are found in the pancreas, liver, and suprarenals; these organs provide substances important in specific regulatory body processes. When experimental rats are deprived of manganese the results are sterility in the male and a lack of maternal instinct in the female. During pregnancy, manganese goes into the blood stream of the unborn child from the mother, and the fecal discharge of the newforn infant contains a remarkable amount. It has been discovered that perosis, a leg-bone deformity in chickens, is accompanied by a manganese deficiency; this may indicate that it plays a similar role in human bone development. Manganese, like many of the other elements, is poisonous to humans in its pure, inorganic form. But in the organic form, as it is found in plants and animals, it is not harmful. Man can only use minerals in the organic form whereas plants use them in the inorganic form.

Both manganese and copper are found only in traces in food, but both accompany iron, and like iron play a part in the manufacture of the blood cells and blood pigment. Evidence indicates that there may be some relationship between copper and the gastric wall. The fact that both are present in varying amounts in all living matter clearly indicates that they are essential for both plant and animal life.

Iron is necessary for the manufacture of hemoglobin molecules which impregnate the red blood corpuscles and give them their red color. The major food sources of iron are of meat and vegetable origin. Muscles or viscera organs and egg yolks are particularly high in iron content, while the iron content of vegetables varies greatly depending largely upon the soil in which they are grown. The body stores iron in the liver and uses it as it needs it, however, iron deficiencies are not uncommon. The usual symptom of an iron deficiency is anemia which is caused by a lack of hemoglobin in the blood. The daily need of iron, for an adult, ranges from six to sixteen milligrams. Iron is also found in large quantities in the bone marrow where the blood corpuscles are manufactured. Iron is necessary for healthy blood.

It will be noted that cobalt and copper play an important part in the assimilation of iron. The three work together as a team. The iron requirements are greater for women than for men. This is due to the loss of iron through menstruation and childbirth. Experiments have shown that women have generally a lesser concentration of iron in their blood than men, but when the iron intake is increased, the concentration becomes about the same. The iron available in foods depends greatly upon the amounts of iron available in the soils in which the foods grew. Due to this fact, we find a greater deficiency of iron in people's blood in some localities than in others.

Cobalt plays a part in increasing the number of red cells in the blood and evidence indicates that it may be beneficial in treating certain types of anemia. Cobalt has been found in exceedingly small quantities in most of the body organs with the exception of the pancreas. Some types of anemia only respond to treatment when iron containing salts of cobalt is administered.

Iron, cobalt, and copper are found together in animal products. If the diet is adequate in animal proteins—meat, fish, fowl, liver, eggs and butter—there is little likelihood of one suffering from a deficiency of these minerals.

The iodine content of soils varies greatly. As a result some foods have considerable iodine while some others are totally deficient in this element. It is one of the essential ingredients of the secretion of the thyroid gland. The needs of the body in respect to iodine are considered to be from one to two milligrams daily. However, it is possible for a person to get along without daily intake for quite some considerable lengths of time, for the iodine containing secretions are broken down after they have served their usefulness and the iodine, less that lost in body excretions, is used again. This presumes a store of iodine with which to begin life. Unfortunately, in some regions of the earth, there is not sufficient iodine in the soil and hence in the foods used in those sections to stock the body's storehouse. In these regions the result of this deficiency is so general that they are designated "goiter belts," being so named from one of the most obvious pathological results of this deficiency.

All people are not affected in the same manner by lessened iodine intake. People whose ancestors came from inland regions need somewhat less iodine and other minerals because their bodies have by inheritance adjusted themselves to this lessened supply. It is not known whether the thyroid secretions are less essential to these people or whether the loss of them through the secretions is lessened, so that they conserve better what they have. It is probable that both factors are important. Since there is a great difference in endocrine patterns, both of the individual and of different races of people, it is possible that the other endocrines may assume some of the functions of the thyroid, thus reducing the need for the thyroid secretions. Whatever the mechanism, the fact remains that people whose ancestors lived in Central Europe are not afflicted to the same degree, as regards pathology in the goiter regions of America, as are people whose ancestry had a plentiful supply of iodine and the other sea minerals living in the same sections.

The soluble minerals such as iodine have been leached from the soils to a considerable extent through the centuries. As a result, they are found principally in the sea and to some extent in the soils bordering the sea where the soil becomes replenished by currents of air containing spray, known in those localities as "salt air."

Thyroid troubles are at a minimum in regions where seaweed and sea fish are used as fertilizers, or where the food consists to a large degree of products from the sea. The use of inorganic iodine in the drinking water or in table salt only partially rectifies iodine deficiency. Although enlargement of the thyroid is less commonly seen where this had been done, other diseases of the thyroid are still prevalent, as is shown by the beneficial effect of small amounts of thyroid substances for a multitude of diseases, including dental caries.

Zinc is always found in human tissues in minute amounts, with the largest concentration in the sex organs and thyroid gland, but its exact role in human physiology is not known. Tin is found in many human tissues with the greatest concentration in the suprarenal glands and the liver, brain, spleen and thyroid glands. Certain tin salts are harmful, but organic tin, that is tin taken into the body through natural foods, seems to be essential to health.

Arsenic in the inorganic form is a well-known poison. In the organic form it is proving to be an indispensable element in human nutrition. It is found in traces in most organs of the body but chiefly in the liver. The liver seems to be the storehouse of this element as well as of many of the vitamins and minerals. In times of need the liver releases arsenic to the blood stream. This happens during menstruation and during the fifth and sixth months of pregnancy and also with cancer. Arsenic seems to be indispensable for the normal development of blood cells in that the unborn child is furnished with large quantities. Arsenic is one of those trace minerals which appears to be closely associated with the physiology of man. In just what way it acts is a ponderous question that remains unsolved.

Bromine is one of the most interesting trace minerals, not for what is known about it, but rather for what is not known about it. It is known that in certain mental ailments such as manic-depressive psychoses, normal blood bromine is reduced to approximately half its normal level and remains low until sound mental health is restored. The bromine content of the blood changes during menstruation. The growth-regulating portion of the pituitary gland contains concentrations seven to ten times greater than that of any other organ. There is considerable variation in bromine content of the tissues with age; after forty-five, the amount begans to fall and at seventy-five years of age only a trace remains. These facts clearly suggest many important questions regarding the action and need of bromine for a healthy body.

It is only within the last few years that boron has been recognized as an essential to plant growth The problem lay in the fact that such minute amounts were needed that it was difficult to produce artificial soils without some trace of boron. When it was done it was found that plants could not grow without it even if everything else was supplied. Boron has something to do with the utilization of calcium by the plant. Because of the universal distribution of boron in the soils and in plant life, it is recognized as an essential to animal nutrition, but in just what manner it is utilized by the animal organism is unknown.

Nickel has been found more widely distributed than cobalt in the human tissues and is particularly concentrated in the pancreas, but nothing is known of its physiological function.

Lithium, rubium, caesium, barium, strontium, beryllium, silver, gold, cadmium, silicon, titanium, as well as traces of nearly all the other metals have been found in human tissues. To date nothing is known about the role, if any, that they play in human nutrition.

Every muscle, nerve, gland and drop of blood in your body requires a continuous supply of minerals for proper nourishment. When there is a deficiency in the diet, or faulty assimilation by the body due to malfunctioning body chemistry, minerals may be withdrawn from the bones and teeth and cause further complications. Prolonged deficiencies of minerals such as calcium, phosphorus, iron and iodine may lead to brittle bones, muscle cramps, soft teeth, nervous irritability and goiter, which affects the thyroid gland. The thyroid, being the regulator gland, when deprived of iodine, then throws the entire endocrine system out of order. Although the exact need of the trace minerals has not been established for humans, it is evident that they are necessary for maintaining a healthy body. From time to time new knowledge of the use of the trace minerals is discovered. It seems reasonable to assume that in the future still more knowledge will be obtained. It is also most likely that everything in the earth's crust will eventually be found to play some part in human nutrition. Evidence strongly indicates that living organisms, being a product of nature and a part of nature, use everything the natural environment contains. Knowing that the mineral content of vegetables varies considerably, depending upon the soil in which they are grown, it is advisable, just to be on the safe side, to take a natural mineral supplement. I give my patients mineral tablets which are compounded from kelp, bone flour and iron; these tablets contain all of the minerals and trace minerals. Also, it is a good policy for people to eat more animal proteins and sea foods, the latter containing practically all of the basic minerals and trace minerals known. Minerals are one of the components necessary for life. They work in harmony with other substances to produce and maintain a state of good health.

V. Menacing Foods and Drinks

Sugar—the Curse of Modern Diet

Today everyone in the United States takes for granted and assumes that refined or processed sugar is a natural and very necessary part of the human diet. No meal or snack is complete without sugar in abundance. By weight, sugar accounts for approximately nine per cent of all the food eaten in the United States. It is added to so many common foods today that one often consumes from one to two cups of sugar per day without realizing that he has eaten any. Yet sugar as we know it, refined sugar, is a concoction of the chemist. It is an unnatural food and is of relatively recent origin in history as a major food or important part of the diet. It was not until the last century that sugar became an important part of the American and European diet, and today it is of little or no importance in other parts of the world except for those areas colonized by Europeans. In George Washington's time, refined sugar cost about $2.40 per pound, and at that price the wealthy used it only for very special occasions. Only a century ago the consumption of sugar was 10 pounds per year per person in the United States. In 1958 the per capita consumption of sugar was around 120 pounds which means that every person in the United States, on the average, consumed 120 pounds of sugar. In 1937 consumption was 100 pounds per person annually. So in a period of a little over two decades the increase has been some 20 pounds and each year it is further increasing. The excessive sugar consumption probably accounts for the great increase in degenerative diseases.

First of all, it is necessary to realize that sugar is not a food but a drug. Refined sugar is a modern fabrication that does not exist in nature. Sugar contains no vitamins or minerals or nutritives necessary to insure good health—it is a pure carbohydrate. According to the *Handbook of Nutrition* of the American Medical Association, the present consumption of sugar is dangerous because it crowds out the consumption of nutritive foods that the body must have to function properly. A Mayo Clinic physician, Dr. Russell Wilder, has found that the use of sugar and sugar products leads to a vitamin B deficiency. Dr. D. T. Quigley maintains that every ounce of sugar which is eaten reduces one's ability to resist and fight infection and it is easy to see why when it is realized that sugar is nothing but "empty calories." Recently a group of scientists and medical physicians, carrying on research at the York Peptic Ulcer Research Trust, York, England, reported that sugar in the diet, not stress and strain, is the major cause of peptic ulcers. When it is understood how adversely sugar affects the endocrine glands of the body and thus throws the body into complete chemical imbalance, it is easy to understand how sugar can well be responsible for peptic ulcers, as well as numerous other degenerative diseases. According to recent research carried on by Dr. Callie Mae Coons and Dr. Madelyn Womack of the Agriculture Department's main research center at Beltsville, Maryland, sugar can be added to the list of foods that are greatly suspected in causing degenerative diseases of the heart and arteries. Their experiments also seem to clearly demonstrate that ordinary table sugar plays an important role in the body's production of cholesterol—the fatty acid which is deadly when its concentration becomes abnormally high. It is most likely then, that sugar, and not fat, is the main culprit in causing cholesterol levels to be high. This relationship is most likely indirect. The body must have a normal cholesterol level. The body manufactures cholesterol from almost any foods eaten, but sugar, as will be shown, causes the glands to eventually become unbalanced, and thus the vital body processes that are controlled by the glands begin to function abnormally. Dr. Coons and Dr. Womack also found, that in their experiments with rats, a sugar plus fat diet combination caused the rats to store more of their food intake as surplus body fat. According to the famed Dr. Royal Lee, synthetic sugars in the form of dextrose, corn syrup, and corn sugar favor the development of cancer, disrupt the assimilation of calcium, and definitely cause diabetes in test animals. These are the most common forms of refined sugar used in candy, ice cream, and soft drinks, but all refined sugar, be it cane or beet sugar or what not, has a very harmful effect upon body chemistry.

From time to time we are all confronted by a well-meaning friend who hands us a full page advertisement pointing out the importance and even necessity of sugar in the diet. "What about this," he asks, "sounds logical to me." Every word of these advertisements is true. But let's sit down with our friend and tell him of the truths that are left unsaid.

Now what are the truths that are overlooked by the research scientists mentioned in these advertisements? First of all, they fail to tell you that although sugar raises the blood sugar level faster than any other food, it also drops the blood sugar level more quickly than any other food, and sometimes to dangerously low levels. During this process, certain endocrine glands of the body are called upon to cope with the emergency situation of handling the intake of refined sugar, which undergoes only one change in the blood stream before becoming immediately usable. The glands must quickly convert this excess sugar into glycogen and store it for future use. During this time the blood sugar level goes up and up until the situation is brought under control. Then this group of glands, having become very fatigued and overworked, lessen their normal functioning. This permits the opposing set of glands to overplay their part with a resulting drop in the blood sugar level in a very short time. In the meantime, calcium and phosphorus levels of the blood are also fluctuating. When this imbalance of body chemistry occurs, it is like a pendulum that is set in motion, continuing to swing first to one side and then to the other before stability is once more regained.

A fact of great significance is that the endocrine glands control not only the blood levels, but all of the functions of the body. In fact, without the functioning of the endocrine glands, death ensues. When these glands must meet the emergency caused by the intake of refined sugar, there is no differentiation in their influence on other functions of the body. All of the cells of our body then become the unwilling victims of the overactivity or underactivity of the controlling endocrine glands.

"There are only eighteen calories in a level teaspoonful of sugar." The sugar advertisement presents this as an inducement for those who are dieting. It has been our observation in treating many, many patients for a number of years, that it is not the daily caloric intake which makes people fat, it is rather the type of foods they eat. We have found that nearly all people on a high protein sugar-free diet will attain and maintain the weight that is best suited to their type of structure and height.

Therefore, by eating natural foods we provide our body with all the sugar it needs for maintaining a stable blood sugar level. On such a diet, there will be little fluctuation of this body sugar level, for the endocrine glands of the body will function at a slower and more normal pace, and all the foods will be digested and assimilated in the wellbalanced rhythm that nature planned.

When the Pied Piper plays his fascinating tune of the goodness and wholesomeness of sugar, there are always those who will follow after him.

The sugar mechanism is a very wonderful and remarkable mechanism. It is controlled by the anterior pituitary gland, the pancreatic gland, and the autonomic nervous system. This system can be compared to a system of two electric motors connected by wires and with a relay switch. When the sugar level is normal the switch is open, and both motors run at their normal speed. When the sugar level of the blood is too high the switch is closed, and the pancreatic motor or gland goes faster. When the sugar level of the blood is too low.the switch operates in reverse, and the anterior pituitary motor or gland runs faster.

The pancreatic motor converts sugar to glycogen, which is stored in the liver and in the muscles, thus lessening the blood sugar level. The anterior pituitary hormones convert the glycogen back into sugar. Thus the two motors or glands serve to maintain the correct sugar level of the blood by alternately working slower and faster. This is a most remarkable mechanism when we consider that some part of all food is converted into sugar by the digestive process. The amounts converted depend upon the kind of foods we eat and the quantities, as well as upon the intervals between meals. We also burn up sugar in irregular amounts. When we exercise we burn it up rapidly, and when resting we burn it up slowly. So we see this relay switch is continually changing the speeds of both glands. In spite of this the sugar level of the blood is maintained at 100 milligrams per 100 cc of blood in a normal, healthy person on a correct diet. It is truly a remarkable mechanism, but abuse can and does wreck it.

Man for thousands of years and generations ate only natural foods, and our sugar regulating apparatus was built to work under these conditions so it seldom got out of order. But modern man has so changed his eating habits in the last two or three generations that a great load has been put upon this automatic sugar regulating apparatus. Instead of converting food into sugar, most people eat or drink substances containing sugar which flood the blood in quantities greater than our sugar mechanisms were designed for. Eventually something has to give.

When this mechanism becomes badly impaired we have diabetes, but before that happens we have what is called a dysfunction of the sugar mechanism. At this pre-diabetic phase the mechanism acts as if it had worn gears. The sugar levels of the blood bounce up and down. Right after a meal the sugar level of the blood is high, and the person having this impaired mechanism gets sleepy. If he is trying to do mental work, either at school or at his business, his efficiency is at low ebb. Many school children flunk the subject given the first hour of the afternoon because of this condition. The eleven o'clock class in the morning is even worse for such a person. He gets faint, his attention is not on his studies. He is very apt to flunk the subject studied at this hour also. At lunch time he is ravenous with hunger. He overeats, particularly of desserts, and then he has to bite his lips in order to stay awake afterward.

This is the picture of thousands of children and adults in the pre-diabetic phase of the breakdown of the sugar level maintaining apparatus. This is the reason for coffee breaks, for caffeine raises the sugar level of the blood. When sugar is added to the coffee this effect is multiplied. As this abuse of the sugar mechanism continues, the coffee breaks come at shorter intervals because the higher the sugar level becomes from this artificial stimulation, the lower it drops afterward and the sooner. If one starts the pendulum swinging in one direction, it will swing just as far off center in the opposite direction.

Our Public Health Service has estimated that there are more than ten million diabetics in our country, and Dr. Abrahamson says in his book, *Body, Mind and Sugar,* that there are at least four times that many in the pre-diabetic stage which we have just described.

How does one correct this pre-diabetic condition. By taking as much load as possible away from this sugar controlling mechanism—by eating less carbohydrate and more protein and fat—by not eating any sugar or sugar containing foods except the natural sugars such as fresh fruits and by not drinking coffee.

With the rest thus given the sugar mechanism, the glands have a chance of recovery and the individual has a very good chance of not only escaping diabetes, but also other degenerative diseases.

Naturally, the glandular system has numerous duties to perform besides the maintenance of the normal sugar level in the blood. One of these duties is to maintain the correct calcium-phosphorus levels of the blood. In general, one group maintains the calcium level, while the other controls the assimilation of phosphorus. These materials are obtained from the food if it is possible to do so, otherwise they are obtained from the storehouse of calcium-phosphorus, the hard tissues of the body. The human body is constructed to maintain both a correct sugar level of the blood and a balance between the calcium and phosphorus of the blood. When man, or any other animal, eats refined sugar, it enters the blood stream at a much greater rate than does the sugar obtained from natural foods. This greatly increased tide of sugar causes group two of the tug of war to work at a greater than normal rate. Since these glands also control the assimilation of calcium, the level in the blood is increased to a greater than normal level Following this action, group one, being opposed by group two, decreases its action to a less than normal extent, resulting in a lower than normal phosphorus level. The pressure of this tug of war upon the glands weakens them and can eventually wear them out. It is evident that sugar is one of the most harmful foods, as it causes erratic calcium-phosphorus levels of the blood and this chemical imbalance may lead to degenerative diseases.

As early as 1869 in the first paper presented at the first Annual Meeting of the Pennsylvania State Dental Society, the relationship between the consumption of sugar and the condition of health was stressed. At that time sugar consumption was only a small fraction of what it is today. Yet, over the years, the profession as a whole, has paid very little attention to this problem. Instead, as far as dental decay is concerned a miracle toothpaste or some miracle chemical put in the water has been sought. The results have all been negative. Dental decay and other degenerative ills are on the increase rather than the decrease. The answer is to be found in diet and good body chemistry.

Nearly all of the information connecting sugar with caries available to the profession concerns the local action of sugar and starches in the mouth. A neglected, but important phase of sugar, in relation to tooth decay is the effect it has on the mouth and the body as a whole after it leaves the mouth and enters the digestive system.

Mouth and dental tissues cannot be separated from the rest of the body; the teeth cannot be effectively treated without inquiring into those materials which feed the teeth, the calcium and phosphorus contained in blood, bone and teeth, and the foods that supply these elements. In this research, the relationship of the blood sugar levels to all of these factors is extremely significant.

To understand more about the action of carbohydrate in the body necessitates mention of a detailed physiology. All mammals require carbohydrate because it is the main ingredient of food which is used for energy. To this end 10 per cent of the fats we eat are changed into sugar; 57 per cent of the proteins are capable of being turned into sugar; 100 per cent of the carbohydrates are converted into sugar. From these sources the animal body was intended to get all of its requirements for sugar. The body manufactures sugar from these raw materials.

Most dentists have had the experience of examining the teeth of patients who had diabetes. Following the discovery of the disease and treatment there was a marked change in the dental condition. If you will recall, the incidence of dental decay was markedly decreased following corrective measures for controlling the diabetes. This occurs as the result of the use of insulin alone. However, there are known to be two types of diabetes—diabetes mellitus, the usual type, and diabetes insipidus, supposedly the infrequent type. The former is recognized as being due to a deficiency of the insulin secreting cells of the isles of Langerhans of the pancreas, and the latter as a deficiency of the posterior pituitary gland. Diabetes insipidus is considered to be rare. However, it is found that a deficiency of the posterior pituitary gland, the supposed cause of diabetes insipidus, is common, and to dentists this is particularly important since many cases of severe peridontal disease are associated with a posterior pituitary gland deficiency. Although a deficient posterior pituitary gland does not affect the sugar levels of the blood markedly, it does affect the calcium-phosphorus levels of the blood, which in turn affects the teeth, gums and jaw bones.

When the posterior pituitary glandular deficiency is corrected, the peridontal condition is improved. Some years ago experiments with two groups of patients with severe pyorrhetic problems were carried out by a dentist in a southern state. One group was treated surgically—the other with the biochemical treatment. The latter proved to be much better. The relationship of diabetes to the blood sugar level is well known. The correlation of the treatment of these two types of disease with the incidence of dental decay and the correction of pyorrhetic conditions should, therefore, be just as meaningful, and the relationship of blood sugar levels to dental situations should be clear and looked upon with increasing importance.

It is clear that there is a definite relationship between diet, blood sugar levels, and calcium-phosphorus ratios. The correct and normal blood sugar is exactly 100 mgs. per 100 cc of blood, while the normal calcium-phosphorus level is 2½ parts calcium to one part phosphorus. The ingestion of sugar (sucrose) markedly affects this relation as has been clinically demonstrated. To demonstrate the effects of sucrose upon the blood sugar level, one ounce of sucrose, levulose, and Tupelo honey was administered to a normal male having a normal blood sugar of 100 mg. per 100 cc of blood, who had been under clinical observation for over a year. The results were as follows:

These tests were administered according to the standard glucose tolerance test procedure to a healthy individual having the normal blood sugar. With one ounce of sugar the blood sugar level rose per 100 cc of blood to 123 mg. the first hour, and fell to 83 mg. the third hour, then rose to 108 mg. per 100 cc of blood the fourth hour, dropped to 98 the fifth hour, and at the end of the fifth hour came back to the normal of 100.

Administering the same test with levulose (from natural fruit sugar) the results were as follows: At the end of one hour following the ingestion of one ounce of levulose the blood sugar jumped to 108 mg. per 100 cc of blood; at the end of two hours the blood sugar had reached 112 mg. per 100 cc of blood, then by the fourth hour it fell to 87 mg per 100 cc of blood, and at the end of the fifth hour had reached 92 mg. per 100 cc of blood.

Honey caused the least fluctuation. Using one ounce of Tupelo honey, at the end of the first hour the blood sugar had climbed to 113 mg. per 100 cc of blood; at the end of the second hour it had fallen to 103 mg. per 100 cc, and by the third hour it stabilized at 100 mg. per 100 cc of blood.

The following cases illustrate what can be done with good nutrition:

Case one began with an alarmingly high blood sugar of 222 mgs. per 100 cc of blood, and an abnormal calcium-phosphorus level of 12.6 calcium to 3.25 phosphorus; that is, 5 milligrams excess calcium. The basic diet (no sugar, coffee, alcohol) was prescribed with marked improvement—blood sugar fell to 167 mg. with only 1¾ mgs. excess calcium. However, this was not enough improvement. Next, the patient was administered 1/200 grain of posterior pituitary gland extract and 13/1200 mgs. of estrogen with a resulting 105 mg. of sugar per 100 cc of blood, and only ¾ mgs. of excess calcium. These improved levels were achieved in one month.

Case two began with a blood sugar of 285 mgs. and a normal calcium-phosphorus level. By administering 15 units of insulin and 1/100 mgs. of testosterone in addition to the basic diet, blood sugar was brought to the normal level without altering the already normal calcium-phosphorus level.

Case three began with 103 mgs. of blood sugar with 2¾ mgs. excess calcium. Basic diet plus 1/100 mgs. of testosterone brought some improvement in calcium-phosphorus levels, but caused the blood sugar to rise to 117 mg. Testosterone was not beneficial in this case. Estrogen, 3/1200 mgs., was then administered with good results; normal blood sugar and calcium-phosphorus levels. This patient had had twenty-seven cavities the year preceding systemic treatment for the cause of her dental ills. She started with a considerable excess of calcium and a low usable compound level. She also had fluctuating blood sugar levels, generally being on the high side. Now, eight years later, it can be reported that she has had no further dental decay, that her blood sugar has stabilized at 100, that she has satisfactory calcium-phosphorus ratios, and that she enjoys excellent health.

Case four began with a low blood sugar of 95 and 2½ mg. excess calcium, and a history of approximately twenty cavities per year. On basic diet alone, the blood sugar level rose to normal with only 1½ mg. excess calcium. Finally, excellent results were achieved with basic diet, 3/800 grs. of posterior pituitary gland extract and 1/1200 milligrams of estrogen. Since this patient, 34 years old, began this treatment more than 1½ years ago, he has had no further dental decay or peridontal diseases and, furthermore, he no longer suffers from a symptom of diabetes insipidus, excessive urination, has lost his excess weight, and is now blessed with the finest of health.

In these treatments, the specific therapy was arrived at by means of maintaining a sugar-free diet, making complete and comprehensive blood analyses, and interpretation of anthropometric graphs. In a clinical survey involving eighty-six current patients, it was demonstrated that the majority of them could gain immunity to dental decay on a sugar-free, natural wholesome diet alone.

Teeth and bone are nourished principally by the calcium and phosphorus levels of the blood. These levels are also controlled by the endocrine glands, and a disturbance in the sugar levels also produces a disturbance in the calcium and phosphorus levels.

Calcium and phosphorus are not used separately to form teeth and bone; they are used as a compound. Like all compounds, these ingredients have a definite relationship one to the other. If this relationship is disturbed, the results are either too much phosphorus or too little phosphorus to go with the calcium. Since the compound can be made only with definite proportions of each, there will be an excess or deficiency of phosphorus. It has been established that to have immunity to caries one must have at least a level of 8.7 mgs. of calcium and a level of 3.5 mgs. of phosphorus per 100 cc of blood.

It is better to have more calcium and phosphorous than less provided the same relationship exists as to quantity. It has been found that in the adult, when the calcium level is 2½ times the phosphorus level the proportions are correct. The amount of these correct proportions are referred to as the usable levels of calcium and phosphorus. The usable levels, obtained by multiplying the amounts of each that can be combined, must be 30 or more to provide immunity to dental decay. The usable level is obtained by multiplying the phosphorus level by 2½ to get the calcium level, or by dividing the calcium level by 2½ to get the phosphorus level. Coronal cavities are due to too low a phosphorus level leaving an excess of calcium. Subgingival dental decay occurs with a too low calcium level for the phosphorus level. A high phosphorus level may be responsible for inflammation of the gums, a certain type of peridontal disease.

The sample cases presented illustrate that where diets have been controlled (sugar eliminated) and normal calcium-phosphorus ratios maintained, immunity to dental decay was achieved, while symptoms of other degenerative diseases tended to disappear. Cases one and two show patients with high blood sugars. In the first, no insulin was required to bring this blood sugar level to normal, but a combination of 2/400ths of a grain of posterior pituitary and 11/1200ths mgs. of estrogen did so. The goal was achieved in a month. In the second, insulin alone had not brought the blood sugar level to a satisfactory point for control of the oral structures. With the addition of testosterone and posterior pituitary gland extract, a correct blood sugar level was obtained within four weeks. There are two important things to note here. First, one case needed insulin, the other did not. Second, both cases required posterior pituitary supplement while one case took the male hormone and the other required the female hormone, but in both instances the correct blood sugar and correct calcium-phosphorus levels were achieved with the result that the patients now enjoy excellent health.

The results in cases three and four were achieved through corrected diet and endocrine support, which produced normalization of the blood sugar levels. The correct calcium-phosphorus ratios could not have been achieved without correction of the blood sugar level. Other means of correcting the too high blood sugar, in addition to insulin, are the use of either estrogen or testosterone as noted, and/or posterior pituitary substance. When there is a low blood sugar level there is a choice of several endocrine substances—thyroid, anterior pituitary and surprisingly enough, the correct sex hormone. Either sex hormone, in the right amount for the individual, will result in the correct sugar level. When the blood sugar level is corrected in the proper manner using the correct delicate tools the correct calcium-phosphorus ratio is ultimately achieved and vice versa. Just as the use of x-ray permitted deeper probing for the cause and means of correction for dental ills, the use of blood tests assists diagnosis in the systemic factors underlying degenerative ills. Oral ills are degenerative in nature and it is now certain that the systemic cause of one degenerative disease may well be related to the systemic cause of others.

Since sugar is such a harmful food, it is natural for one to wonder why so little is said about this subject. The answer is perhaps, that the sugar industry is exceptionally wealthy and powerful, and controls much of the research done with regard to sugar. Foundations financed and controlled by major processed food corporations and sugar industries each year grant money to universities for research. But, they control the projects that are to be investigated and although much valuable research has been accomplished, nothing is ever found wrong with sugar.

Sugar is included in so many foods today, that it is wise to read the labels and note that it may be listed as sugar added, dextrose, light syrup, or heavy syrup. Everyone knows that the basic ingredient of candy is sugar and is a major ingredient of cookies, cakes, pies, ice cream and prepared desserts in general. Sugar is also generally added to most frozen and canned fruits, (so much so that their natural flavor is lost), to many processed meats, luncheon meats, wieners, frankfurters, commercial whole wheat breads, pancake mixes, bread mixes, peanut butter, soft drinks, many kinds of cocktails and numerous other commercial foods. Even chewing gum consists of 50 to 75 per cent sugar. A natural, wholesome diet eliminates all refined or processed sugar and all commercial foods that contain sugar. Only pure, unpasteurized honey and genuine black strap molasses can be used safely, but they must be used in moderation. Even fruits, which are wholesome foods, should be eaten in moderation. The body can be overloaded with natural sugar. Refined sugar is such a harmful food, being a major factor in causing degenerative ills, that it may well be the one food that could lead us to a nation of physically sick people. Statistics today show that degenerative ills are increasing at an alarming rate and are attacking people at an ever increasingly earlier age. It is time that the fact be recognized that diet is largely responsible for this increase and that sugar is one of the major culprits.

Artificial Sweeteners

What are artificial sweeteners? What does it mean when food products are marked "artificially sweetened"? It means that a chemical, a synthetic substance fabricated in a laboratory, having no nutritive value, no calories, and which is actually a drug, is the substance used. The artificial sweeteners commonly used today are saccharin (a coal-tar crystaline product), sodium saccharin, sodium cyclamate, calcium cyclamate, or potassium cyclamate. Some of these drugs, labeled as artificial sweeteners, go under the regular chemical names while others are marketed under various trade names.

There are a number of reasons why artificial sweeteners should not be used. Man has four tastes—sweet, salt, sour, and bitter. The taste buds are located on the tongue and are intended by nature to be guides in selecting good, wholesome food. Artificial sweeteners will satisfy the sense of taste for sweet but will not satisfy the metabolic needs of the body for natural, wholesome carbohydrates. Artificial sweeteners are more than just "empty calories," such as sugar and refined starches, they are complete drugs with no food value whatsoever. Dietary habits begun in childhood or later, can be badly distorted by excessive use of sugar, sugar products, and artificial sweeteners. They build up a dependence upon sweet things and lead to the belief that sweetness should normally be expected in many foods, instead of realizing that it is an exceptional taste in the basic foods to which man's digestive mechanism has become adapted over thousands of years. Unfortunately, the digestive tracts of man do not change to meet the new offerings of the supermarket shelves and freezers. Man's digestive tract is just the same as it was 10,000 years ago. The human digestive tract was not constructed to handle drugs such as artificial sweeteners; or, as a matter of fact, refined sugar (and this includes brown sugar and raw sugar as well as white "sugar bowl" sugar).

Artificial sweeteners act as irritants upon the taste buds and thus give the false sensation of sweetness. Anyone who has used too much of them will complain of a bitter taste in the mouth. These chemicals are so constructed that they irritate or prick the sweet taste buds and thus give the sensation of sweetness when taken in a very small amount. When you use artificial sweeteners, you are using a false or fake sweetener which really irritates and deceives the taste buds into thinking that they taste sweetness. Continued use of these, as well as sugar, dulls the sensitivity of the taste buds to natural sweetness so that one cannot really enjoy the true and wholesome sweetness of fruits or other naturally sweet foods. That is why many people want sugar or an artificial sweetener added to canned fruits and fresh fruits. When one has not dulled his taste

for natural sweetness, the full flavor of fruit is very deli-
cious and just right with that distinctive flavor characteristic of each fruit. When a person has been accustomed to
artificial sweeteners and refined sugars, it usually takes
about three to four weeks for him to regain his natural
taste for sweetness after having dispensed with the use of
these drugs and/or sugar.

The most important reason for not using artificial sweeteners is that their safety, and particularly that of the cyclamates, has not been fully verified or established. It is
well known that the cyclamates do unfavorably affect the
intestinal tract, but as of the present date, medical research has established a probability that they are actually
harmful and they are being removed from the market.
Many of the synthetic sweeteners such as saccharines, are
made from coal tar crystalline products, which are poisonous and very much suspected by scientists as cancer causing substances. Many of the food dyes used are also coal
tar dyes and fall in the same category with the synthetic
sweeteners in being highly suspected as playing a part in
causing cancer. A food coloring usually called butter yellow was used for several years before it was discovered
that it caused cancer of the liver. It is no longer used.
Most people are not even aware of the fact that practically
all dairy butter is colored to make it uniform, however, the
coloring agents are supposed to be harmless. Standards
have been set up for a number of products and all are supposed to conform by law to that standard. As these standards are set, the ingredients are not listed on the package.
One of these is ice cream. The standards permit ice cream
to contain the stabilizer sodium carboxymethyl-cellulose,
(which makes for smoothness), coal-tar dyes and artificial
flavoring agents. The famed Dr. Hueper of the Food and
Drug Administration has named the first of these substances as a cancer causing suspect, while the coal-tar
derived food additives are also suspected of causing the
same degenerative disease. Other sweeteners, which were
once considered to be perfectly safe and harmless, were
later found to be very definitely injurious to health. In one

instance a commercial sugar substitute, Dulcin, which had been in use for over fifty years and considered to be perfectly safe, was found to have the capacity of adversely affecting blood and causing large liver tumors in rats; so reports William Longgood in his book, *The Poisons in Your Food*. Today most of the experts are of the scientific opinion that both the cyclamates and saccharins should be under careful observation for long periods of time to determine any ill effects which may develop from their use. People on a salt free diet (which is not necessary when you have good body chemistry) should be advised that some artificial sweeteners contain sodium which is salt even though the sodium content may not be listed on the label.

The best way to curtail the use of sweets is just to stop eating them and eat fruits and natural sweets in moderation. There is no healthful artificial sweetener; and, in that they are synthetic drugs, their continued use may possibly be very injurious to health. They dull the true sense of taste just as refined sugar does and thus prevent one from enjoying natural flavor as created by nature. Artificial sweeteners and artificially sweetened foods should be avoided if sound body chemistry is to be maintained.

Milk—the not so perfect food

Over the past few decades we have been increasingly led to believe that milk is indispensable to sound health. The propaganda on the essentiality of milk has been so intensive that it comes as something of a shock when we hear that milk is not necessary to good health and may be detrimental to sound health. The high pressure advertisements on the good effects of milk drinking remind one of the old statement which declares, that if you state something long enough, loud enough, and persistently enough, people will come to believe it without ever questioning the soundness or basis from which such a statement was derived. It seems that this is largely true of milk. From the cradle to the grave, we hear "drink your milk" for good health, sound teeth and bones—and we do that even though our teeth keep on decaying, our bones may get brittle and we have colds and diseases right along. Obviously, milk is not as healthful a food as the public has been led to believe. But first, before examining what many authorities have to say about the effects of milk, let us see just what milk is.

Before a child is born, the developing child is provided with oxygen for breathing and ready-to-use food materials for growth from the mother's blood. Following birth, the infant breathes itself, but it still must have nutritive materials from its mother, which are supplied in the form of her milk. Actually, the mother's milk replaces the blood by which the infant was formerly fed. Milk resembles blood; it is blood without the respiratory substances, that is, the red blood cells and blood pigment. For this reason milk may be aptly described or termed white blood, because that is exactly what it is. Each mammal produces milk for its young and it is different from that of every other milk-producing species of animal, just as their blood is different. The milk produced by each species of animals, such as humans, dogs, horses and cows is designed by nature for its young. Milk is supposed to be used for only a limited period, which is until the young have developed sufficiently to eat regular foods. All animals know when that time has arrived, and with humans, this occurs when the baby begins to grow teeth and it becomes uncomfortable for the mother to nurse the child—the bite of the baby's teeth hurt. This signifies that milk should be withdrawn from the diet and the child should then commence eating solid foods of a wholesome nature so that he will grow healthy and strong.

We are a nation of drinkers of cow's milk which is intended by nature for a calf, not for human consumption. Cow's milk is entirely different from human milk. To begin with, a calf is a much coarser creature than a human baby and thus cow's milk is correspondingly more coarsely composed. When cow's milk is examined with an ultramicroscope, the molecules of protein show up as hazy spots of light, while those of human milk are not as easily seen because the groups of human milk protein are much finer. A difference can also be noted in its action in the human stomach. When a child has been fed cow's milk, cheese clumps form in the stomach and when a child vomits, cheese is what he expels. On the other hand, when a child who has been fed human milk vomits, only fine flakes appear.

The milk of each animal species contains growth hormones in a concentration suitable for the developmental requirements of the young of the species. These growth hormones are secretions of the anterior pituitary gland which promote and control growth. Naturally, as one can see, the growth hormones of different species of animals vary greatly. For example, a rabbit completely doubles its original weight at birth in six days, a dog in nine days, a sheep in fourteen days, a goat in twenty-two days, a cow in forty-seven days, a horse in sixty days, and man doubles his weight from birth in one hundred and eighty days. It has previously been pointed out that these growth hormones, in fact all hormones secreted by the endocrine glands, are like powerful little hydrogen bombs. It is easy to surmise what effect the growth hormones of a cow, which are a major ingredient of the cow's milk, might do to a human. Some people think that the over-consumption of milk may account for so many Americans growing so tall, yet not particularly noted for excellent health. The growth hormones of the cow act upon the human child when he drinks milk. If he is born with an overactive anterior pituitary gland, then he is getting a double dose or more, so to speak, of growth stimulant which may result in his growing to be excessively tall and skinny—the beanstalk type. These hormones added to what the body usually produces for itself after passing through the nursing or infant stage, may throw the individual's body into such a chemical imbalance as to bring about disaster.

There may possibly be a correlation between certain types of cancer and a large consumption of cow's milk. It has been noted for well over a decade that the incidence of specific types of cancer occur primarily in those regions and countries where the consumption of cow's milk is very high and constitutes a major part of the diet. In that cancer is largely cells gone crazy—cells that grow more rapidly than the normal healthy cells of the body—it may well be that such a condition may be promoted by constantly taking into the body the growth hormones that are intended by nature to promote growth in a calf, not a human. Today, this problem may be even more acute because milk cows have become something of freaks. In an effort to get cows to produce more and more milk for a longer and longer period of time, cows have been bred and developed to have greatly overactive pituitary glands. This, of course, is evidenced in the milk they produce. These growth hormones are contained in the protein of the milk and according to Maynard Murray, M.D., are not affected by boiling, pasteurization, or cooking. Therefore, they are not only found in milk, but in all milk products, such as cheese. This does not include heavy cream and butter. They are animal fats which merely come with the milk, therefore one is safe in using these products. That is why we recommend substituting heavy cream for milk; for one cup of milk, substitute ⅓ cup of heavy cream diluted with ⅔ cup of water.

Cow's milk also differs in many other respects from that of human milk. Seventy-seven per cent of the phosphorus in human milk is in the form of organic compounds most similar to those of the human body, whereas only twenty-eight per cent of the phosphorus compounds found in cow's milk are of an organic type. A child's body must make a much stronger effort to utilize the phosphorus of cow's milk than is the case with human milk, where any effort that is needed is easy and natural. This situation may be illustrated as follows. Each child must have building blocks for its body. The blocks it gets from cow's milk are too large and cumbersome and must be cut down, to the right size. However, from its mother's milk, the child gets blocks which are just the right size and can be used immediately.

Many years ago, Dr. I. M. Rabinowitch, then director of the Metabolism Department of Montreal General Hospital, said that the dairy industries would like us to flood our bodies with milk. He asks if milk is actually an indispensable part of the adult human's diet? The answer is "no." Briefly, milk is given by the mammalian adult to its young and varies in different animal species from almost one month to approximately one year after birth. Hence, no animal in the state of nature is furnished with milk after weaning. Thus it is obvious that milk is not a natural food for the adult animal. Since these animals live and continue to reproduce, one can readily see that the adult diet contains all of the necessary food elements which are supplied in the maternal milk. Man is no different from the other animals with regard to diet as adapted to his needs for health.

Milk has been proven to be an incomplete food even for young animals. Only after a few months of age, calves must be given mineral supplements in their feeding or else they are likely to die of anemia. Also, the rapidity with which this unhealthy condition will progress depends upon the quantity of milk consumed, because milk is not an adequate food for supplying the needs of the blood-building organs of the body. This has been proven experimentally with the use of rats.

Dr. J. Sim Wallace, an outstanding medical and dental scientist, in his book *The Physiology of Oral Hygiene*, states that where the land flows with milk and sugar, there you have dental decay rampant in the classes which eat these foods most, notwithstanding their vitamin content. It would seem that by this time dieticians might know that the hygiene of the mouth is not maintained by milk, bread soaked in milk, milk desserts and milk and crackers. These and many other foods falling in the same category, are examples of the things that should not be recommended by anyone who desires healthy teeth and good oral hygiene.

Many years ago medical men began making reference to the undue emphasis placed on milk that was mainly based on limited experiments with animals. Dr. William Dock, an outstanding specialist in the field of coronary disease, has noted that though young Japanese men have been accustomed to long hours of physical labor, they are relatively immune to atherosclerosis and coronary disease which is becoming increasing more prevalent, and alarmingly so, in the United States. The Japanese drink no milk, and Dr. Dock believes this to be one of the reasons for their immunity to these two degenerative heart diseases.

Recent research is proving Dr. Dock to be correct in suspecting milk as a cause of heart and circulatory diseases. Medical research investigators at the Washington University School of Medicine carried on a study of hundreds of autopsy reports and clinical records of ten hospitals in the United States and five in England from 1940 to 1959. The results of this significant medical research showed that in the United States, the prevalence of heart attacks was more than twice as high among people who were heavy milk drinkers than it was among non-milk drinkers. For Great Britain the results were practically the same. A complete report on the findings of this very important research has been published by the American Heart Association in the April, 1960 edition of *Circulation*.

Dr. H. M. Sinclair, Vice-President of Magdalenia College, Oxford University and an eminent British researcher in nutrition, has long recognized the inferiority of cow's milk and the tendency to overfeed children with milk. Dr. Sinclair believes that excessive feeding of milk during the period when the child is growing is not desirable, and may lead to early maturity which within itself will lead to untimely death due to chronic degenerative diseases. In other words, overfeeding during the growing period of children shortens this period, brings adult size quicker, and shortens life. Excessive rapid growth of children in the United States, where overfeeding of milk is common, may very likely hasten the development of such chronic degenerative diseases as heart disease, kidney disease, and even cancer.

Doctors Harold D. Lyncn and W. D. Snively, Jr., at an American Medical Association Meeting in Minneapolis, noted that beverages, including milk and juices, can be poured down a baby's throat fairly easily, whereas those foods high in protein, which must be eaten if a child is to grow healthy, are not sweet and must be chewed. It would appear that children quickly become conditioned to those foods which require little effort to eat, and consequently learn to prefer the soft, liquid, sweet foods. They are thus robbed of good nutrition (high protein foods, such as meat, poultry, fish, and other foods that must be chewed) and therefore build no resistance to dental decay and infectious disease.

Amy L. Daniels and Gladys Everson, nutritionists at the State University of Iowa, noted in a paper on poor appetite in pre-school children, that many children are overfed on milk, often causing symptoms of anemia, constipation, and vitamin deficiencies (milk does not contain all of the necessary vitamins). Dr. Eugene Rosamond, when addressing a state pediatric and regional medical society meeting. said that a quart of milk per day for each child was excellent commercial propaganda, but poor medical advice. He also said that approximately seven per cent of all sick children who go to the physician are ailing because their mothers are requiring them to drink more milk than they need. He further estimates that ten per cent of the minor ills of children are due to the evils of too much milk, and agencies and organizations that promote the betterment of the welfare of children have circulated the slogan of a quart of milk a day for each child so that mothers feel that the authority of the United States Government is in support of this advice. Children need good solid food—meat, eggs, fish, fresh vegetables and fruits—in order to be healthy. Dr. Rosamond lists the following typical symptoms of too much milk in the diet of children: pallor from anemia, constipation, irritability on the part of the child, refusal to eat (and the mother usually insists on more milk), restless sleeping, bad dreams, bed-wetting, and in some cases even a morbid appetite for abnormal substances such as dirt. In the Journal of the American Dental Association, Dr. J. Sim Wallace wrote back in 1935, that dieticians seem to forget that when an infant reaches the age of two and one-half years, its digestive apparatus has been altered from one end to the other, and the milk which was needed in early infancy is no longer necessary nor desirable for the physiological development of the jaws, teeth, and alimentary canal generally. Children should have solid food. They should not be filled with milk, juices and sweets.

For years the dairy industry has gone all out to popularize milk and hence increase its consumption to the greatest possible extent. One of their major slogans states that people never outgrow their need for milk, and should drink three glasses of milk every day. A large group of Yale students took this advice seriously and some even went on milk binges. This prompted the University's Department of Public Health to warn that the normal healthy individual can readily cause kidney stone formation by simply drinking or eating too much milk.

Too much calcium in the system can create toxic effects upon the body. Dr. Mark Hegsted of the Harvard School of Public Health, stated that there has been an overemphasis on calcium in nutrition and that this, closely tied to the urging of everyone to consume great quantities of milk, may have harmed the health of the adolescent and adult population. For thirty years or more, dieticians and nutritionists have persistently urged increased, lifelong milk consumption because of the alleged need of each person for a high calcium intake, but medical experts hold that an excess of calcium may probably produce an undesirable effect on the kidneys, causing, for example, the formation of kidney stones. Dr. Philip H. Henneman noted that kidney stones are often found in people who drink a quart of milk per day, and further found that they had no further development of kidney stones following the discontinuance of milk. Dr. Prien, Assistant Professor of Urology at the world-famous Boston University School of Medicine, made a complete examination of 1,000 kidney stones and found that ninety per cent of them contained calcium. Dr. Prein thinks that the eating of too much calcium, that is, foods that contain very high amounts of calcium such as milk and cheese, may be a factor in causing kidney stones.

Government nutritional experts have recommended 800 milligrams of calcium daily for the average adults; however, on the basis of recent research, specialists believe that only 150 milligrams per day is sufficient. The Journal of the American Medical Association recognizes that many of the allowances of the Food and Nutrition Board of the National Research Council may be excessive. Dr. E. M. Nelson, the late distinguished director of the Division of Nutrition of the United States Food and Drug Administration, stated in a paper which appeared in Food Facts and Fallacies in 1959, that the evidence in the recommended dietary allowance for calcium is very much too high. People do not have to drink milk or eat cheese to get calcium; calcium is supplied in abundance in many foods that we eat daily and is found in most vegetables and fruits. For example, the calcium content of the following foods is as follows:

2 ounces salmon: 112 mg.
5 oysters: 95 mg.
2 ounces shrimp: 69 mg.
8 large olives: 101 mg.
6 figs: 223 mg.
5 clams: 100 mg.
1 cup broccoli: 130 mg.
cup beet greens: 118 mg.

Nuts, beans, cauliflower, sea food, and hard water are also very rich in calcium. From the limited list given above, it is easy to see that one does not need to drink milk and eat cheese in order to get enough calcium.

Calcium is necessary for the conduction of nerve impulses; it forms a necessary element in the cement that binds cells together in body tissue; it plays a part in keeping the heart beat normal; and is essential for healthy bones and teeth. It is natural to ask where one will get enough calcium if he does not drink milk and eat milk products. First of all, it takes only a small amount of calcium for the system to perform these vital functions, and too much puts a burden upon the system. Calcium absorption of the body is controlled by the endocrine glands, and the body can get all of the calcium it needs from a natural, wholesome diet.

Most of the people of the world do not drink milk after they have been weaned by their mother. The Chinese react to drinking milk with complete disgust; their reaction is the same as ours when someone mentions drinking and eating blood. There is some similarity in the two reactions because milk is merely white blood—the Chinese react to both with equal disgust. The American Indians, many African Negro tribes, large groups of the Asiatic people and the Polynesians never drink milk after they have been weaned, yet these people are healthy and strong, and show no deficiency in calcium whatsoever. Dr. A. R. P. Walker of the famed South African Institute for Medical Research found that although it is assumed that large amounts of calcium are essential to pregnant women and nursing mothers, such probably is not true. He found that Bantu women, who get very little calcium in their diet and never drink milk, produce a much higher quality of breast milk than do British and American mothers. Anthropological studies of primitive peoples and of other civilizations clearly prove that milk, after weaning, is not necessary or even desirable. Most of these primitive peoples, such as the Polynesians, Maya Indians, and Eskimos, who never drink milk, are remarkably healthy on their native diet, and dental decay is a rarity among them. Certainly this indicates that milk cannot, and does not, stop dental decay. On the contrary, Dr. Brunn of Denmark, an outstanding dentist who has spent years in research checking the oral condition of children of Denmark, England, Sweden, Switzerland, and South America, finds that in the mouths of children who drank milk, the residue left by the milk forms a cheese around the teeth and crevices. This mouth cheese is probably a factor in causing dental decay.

Because of the excessive amount of calcium in milk and the animal hormones, cow's milk, in time, can upset the calcium-phosphorus levels of the body. When the calcium and phosphorus level is affected adversely, body chemistry is off balance with the result that the mouth may become acid. Bacteria thrives in an acid medium, and thus the drinking or taking of cow's milk and milk products again is a factor in causing dental decay as it may play a part in assisting the mouth to become an incubator for harmful bacteria to grow and thrive.

In an article which appeared in Medical Science, January 2, 1957, Dr. Harold D. Lynch, an outstanding pediatrician, stated that the consumption of one quart of milk per day, without attention to solid protein foods, definitely encourages dental decay. Dr. Lynch further noted that children who drink large quantities of milk also develop a tendency to eat large amounts of sweets and starches. Milk is not an adequate source of protein, and protein is the governing nutrient for growing children. Dr. Alfred S. Schwarts, Assistant Professor of Clinical Medicine, Washington University, has pointed out that severe nutritional anemia is more common among children who use large quantities of milk.

Now that we are living in the atomic age, with the detonation of so many atomic and hydrogen bombs in experiments, the atmosphere is becoming contaminated with Strontium 90 which, when it reaches a certain level in the body, can be fatal. Strontium 90 is a bone-seeking substance which, after many years, may cause leukemia or cancer and, therefore, its intake into the body should be kept at the lowest possible level. Presently, milk seems to be the main source by which Strontium 90 is entering the body. Radioactivity in milk doubled in Great Britain in the spring of 1955, and it is rapidly increasing everywhere in the world.

Some authorities, such as Dr. W. O. Caster of the Department of Physiological Chemistry at the University of Minnesota, have recommended that milk processors should treat milk to remove the calcium where the Strontium 90 is stored. (Ironically enough, the calcium content of milk is the very reason why many nutritionists have long advocated increased consumption of milk by everyone.) We, here at the Page Foundation, think one of the simplest solutions is to stop drinking milk. You who are familiar with Dr. Page's work will recall that for years he has been advocating that milk from a cow is an unnatural food for a human adult, and probably interferes with the establishment of good body chemistry. It is encouraging to note that specialists in many branches of the healing arts, and in research relating to such, are also beginning to realize that milk is not such a healthy food after all.

Often penicillin and other antibiotic residues are present in milk. These may cause unfavorable reactions in persons who are allergic to antibiotics, and it may further build up a resistance to the effectiveness of antibiotics when they are needed during serious illness. Dr. Murray C. Zimmerman reported in the American Medical Association Archives of Dermatology in 1959 that penicillin reactions which have produced death are greatly increasing. Dr. Zimmerman, an authority in the field of medicine, thinks that the increase may be due to allergies that are precipitated by the daily consumption of milk and milk products. Penicillin is often used to treat mastitis, a common disease which attacks the cow's udder. For this reason a high percentage of milk and dairy products are contaminated. A spot-check of 1700 grocery store samples of milk from 48 states and the District of Columbia was made by the Food and Drug Administration in 1957 and 11 per cent of the milk checked was found to be contaminated with measurable residues of penicillin. Anywhere from 5 to 12 per cent of all milk samples tested by the Food and Drug Administration have been found to contain harmful residues of antibiotics.

Due to large scale publication of the harmless effects of DDT and similar pesticides widely used, most people believe that it is not poisonous to humans. However, it is tremendously poisonous. It is a cumulative poison, and when a certain point is reached in the body, serious illness may result. In 1958 a survey conducted by the Food and Drug Administration indicated that eleven large cities across the nation were being supplied with milk that contained substantial amounts of chemical insect killers; these pesticides were DDT and other chemical agents containing chlorine. Although it is strictly against the law for DDT and other dangerous chemical pesticides to be present in milk, it has been reliably estimated that at least half and probably more, of all the commercial milk distributed to consumers contains DDT or other poisonous pesticide residues.

When milk is exposed to the air, it forms a perfect medium for bacteria or germs to flourish. Fortunately, most bacteria are harmless, some are helpful to man, but others such as tuberculosis, undulant fever germs, etc., are very harmful and can cause death. Milk largely becomes contaminated with bacteria by being exposed to air. Milk, intended for babies by nature, is never exposed to air. The infant or baby takes milk directly from the mother into the mouth and swallows it. The general public has been led to believe that pasteurization kills the bacteria in milk. This is largely true immediately following pasteurization, but then as time passes the bacteria begin to grow again and the number of bacteria in pasteurized milk increases by the thousands as the hours pass. This can be verified by merely having a bacteria culture test run on the pasteurized milk delivered to your door. The results will probably startle you. One authority, Dr. Maynard Murray, has characterized pasteurized milk as a "bacteria soup" because when the bacteria are killed by pasteurization the dead bacteria are left in the milk. As these dead bacteria decay, they build up toxic or poisonous substances which can, if the concentration gets strong enough, cause sickness.

Obviously, milk is not nature's perfect food as the general public has been led to believe. For the infant prior to the weaning age, when taken as intended by nature, it is necessary. But milk for children and adults is not a desirable food.

Although there has been a great deal of quackery in the fields of food and nutrition, there has been lots of quackery which has escaped criticism because it is approved and accepted by important interests. According to an article in the prestigious *Consumers' Bulletin,* the chief organizations which misinform the public with regard to food and nutrition are a large number of commercial and governmental agencies that constantly advocate and propagate the necessity of providing large quantities of milk in the diet for young and old alike.

Coffee, Tea, Tobacco and Alcohol

Today there are a number of stimulants commonly in wide usage which can and do have a harmful effect upon body chemistry. Stimulants are substances that are taken into the body, not for their nutritive qualities, but because they exert some desired effect on the nervous system. The most prevalent and harmful of these stimulants is coffee. Coffee is a beverage which came into common and general use only in the modern era. The appreciation of coffee as a beverage in Europe dates from the latter part of the 17th century and the early colonist brought the custom to America. However, it was used only as a luxury item and in strict moderation. Coffee originated in Ethiopia, and it was the Ethiopians who discovered that it made an effective stimulating beverage. From them it passed to the Arabs, and hence on to Europe. As long as coffee is used very moderately and only occasionally, its harmful effects are not so great; but when it becomes a constant habit and is consumed many times daily, coffee is likely to have very harmful effects. The general hereditary constitution of the individual concerned is the factor that makes the time element short or long.

Many people wonder why coffee is harmful and must be avoided if good body chemistry is to be attained and maintained. The culprit in coffee is caffeine, a substance related chemically to uric acid. Let's see what caffeine does to one's body chemistry. Caffeine is a stimulant, so when you drink a cup of coffee, the caffeine stimulates the adrenal cortex to produce more of its hormones; this in turn induces the liver to break down glycogen (body stored sugar) into glucose (sugar), which flows into the blood stream. This is the explanation why a cup of coffee "gives you a lift." However, it is really an artificially induced lift and trouble develops because the isles of Langerhans of the pancreas, which produce insulin, cannot tell the difference between the effects of drinking coffee and eating food. They don't know whether the sugar has come from the food that is being digested or from previously stored glycogen which has been broken down by the action of the caffeine's stimulus on the adrenal cortex. The isles of Langerhans go to work to force the blood sugar to its normal level and, in the course of time, because of their repeated stimulation due to drinking coffee, the isles of Langerhans become so sensitive that they over-respond to normal stimulation. This gradually, but progressively, breaks down their efficiency. According to E. M. Abrahamson, M.D., a noted specialist on diabetes and hyperinsulinism, caffeine is a major causative factor in certain kinds of depression, which may be regarded as a form of caffeine poisoning. He states that one of the major reasons for the widespread condition of hyperinsulinism in the United States is due to excessive consumption of caffeine.

It has been noted that there is evidently a relationship between the ingestion of caffeine and sugar and peptic ulcers. On a percentage basis, the service men in World War I had fewer incidences of ulcers than those of World War II and, likewise, the combat troops of World War II had a much smaller percentage of peptic ulcers than those in the camps. The explanation seems to be that when in combat, the troops got less coffee and sugar.

Only a few decades ago, Americans were accustomed to a good, healthy breakfast of eggs, bacon, ham, grits or potatoes, but now we are city dwellers and go in for a very light breakfast. For breakfast many people fortify themselves only with black coffee and cigarettes and, of course, they get an immediate lift as their glands are overworked

to put the blood sugar up and/or stimulate the nervous
system. But remember, it is a lift produced by a stimulant,
by artificial means. That is why they begin to feel fatigued
around 10 a.m.; but the coffee break takes care of that
until lunch, then some food and more coffee—another
coffee break at mid-afternoon, coffee on arriving home
and then at dinner. You can see that the person is being
constantly pushed along by the stimulation of caffeine.
Eventually, following such a course year after year, can
lead to, or be a major factor in causing numerous degenerative processes. It wears the glands out by keeping the
blood sugar level jumping up and then down in the body's
efforts to maintain a normal blood sugar level.

Many people who are trying to lose weight drink black
coffee to dull the pangs of hunger and still have pep, but
they are merely making the situation worse. As you can
see, this repeated stimulus to the isles of Langerhans resulting in low blood sugar, makes them even more sensitive, makes the rigid diet more difficult because the coffee's appetite-quenching qualities become increasingly
briefer and are followed by a ravenous appetite. Many people just drink more coffee when this happens and thus re-
peat the cycle and steadily and rapidly wear out their glands
by overworking them.

In addition to having a most adverse effect upon the
glands, coffee also stimulates the nerve cells. Controlled
clinical tests that I have closely supervised showed a
marked lowering in blood sugar when coffee was taken,
yet the individuals felt fresh with an abundance of energy.
The effect, as described by one person who is not a coffee
drinker and hence has not built up a tolerance for coffee,
stated that it was like a small dose of benzedrine, the main
ingredient of a very dangerous drug that many people
have taken for quick energy, to stay awake, or to reduce.
Coffee increases the pulse rate and the amplitude of the
heartbeat; it also increases the tonus of the skeletal muscles. Coffee causes a more active secretion of the gastric
glands with the result that people who suffer from too

much gastric secretion often suffer from heartburn after drinking coffee. Experts agree that coffee is particularly harmful for people who suffer from ulcers. In that coffee increases the digestive juices in the stomach which are responsible for continued irritation, it is obvious that coffee plays a part in preventing healing. Renal activity is increased by drinking coffee so that large amounts of salts are taken from the blood. Coffee can be a poison for laboratory animals when they drink it in large quantities over a long period of time. It is well known that it can produce poisonous effects in small children. Nervous people are made more nervous by drinking coffee, which merely aggravates the situation. The characteristic symptoms of too much coffee drinking are palpitation of the heart, headaches, insomnia, nervousness, and digestive trouble. Coffee is known to destroy vitamin C in the body so that coffee drinkers may be deficient in this vital vitamin which is necessary for healthy tissue and to ward off infectious diseases.

In 1959 the per capita consumption of coffee was 16 pounds; that means that for every man, woman and child in the United States, 16 pounds of raw coffee were used. When this 16 pounds of coffee is added to water to make the beverage, you can only imagine how many gallons of coffee were consumed. Like sugar, coffee consumption is on the increase and with this increase, it is likely that degenerative diseases will also increase, as coffee has a most harmful effect upon body chemistry.

Tea is another stimulating beverage which contains caffeine and tannic acid which is hard on the kidneys. Actually, one cup of medium strong tea contains the same amount of caffeine as a regular cup of coffee, but it does not stimulate nearly as much in that caffeine, to give maximum stimulation, must be combined with other substances which are found in coffee but lacking in tea. Tea should be used only moderately and then in very weak form.

People who wish to maintain good body chemistry, which is synonymous with good health, should eliminate from their diet beverages that contain the alkaloid of caffeine. The caffeine-containing beverages or foods are listed as follows: coffee, tea, soft drinks that contain caffeine, cocoa and chocolate.

From this brief resume of the effects of coffee upon the body chemistry, it is easy to conclude that coffee, as well as the other things containing caffeine, should be deleted from one's diet. Coffee has no nutritive value; it may be characterized as a stimulant which overworks the glands and can eventually wear them out with the result that degenerative disease may become prevalent within the body. When sugar and milk are added to coffee, that merely makes it a more difficult beverage for the body to handle; it is like "burning the candle at both ends" as far as maintaining body efficiency and health are concerned.

Tobacco is another substance commonly used that falls within the modern age. When America was discovered, Europeans found the Indians inhaling, usually from a pipe, the smoke from the burning leaves of a plant called tobacco. However, the Indians used it ceremonially and very moderately. From this modest beginning, smoking has become a national characteristic. Smoking signifies that a boy or girl has grown up, and all manner of psychological attachments are associated with the smoking complex. The use of tobacco may be described as a national addiction and is becoming widespread in most civilized societies. Each year the consumption of tobacco increases and along with it certain degenerative diseases increase, which add mounting proof that smoking is not a healthful habit. In addition to nicotine, tobacco smoke contains a number of very poisonous gases such as hydrocyanic acid, pyridine, the deadly poisonous hydrogen disulphide, ammonia—which causes irritation to the mucous membranes and causes smoker's catarrh—and a number of other gases. Actually, a cigar contains so much poison that it would kill two men if they were to take its complete contents into the body. Fortunately, smokers take only a small amount of these gases into the system; but over a period of years this is, no doubt, bound to have a very harmful effect upon the body.

Many people say that they smoke to reduce appetite and thus not gain excessive weight. It is true that smoking does inhibit the production of gastric juices, but this is not a very sound way to approach the problem of reducing.

Nicotine has a decided effect upon the system. The nicotine which enters the blood stream from the lungs and circulates in the blood, paralyzes the ganglia, or "switchboards," of the sympathetic nervous system. The action of nicotine is antagonistic to adrenalin, the hormone of the adrenal gland which inhibits the normal movements of the intestines. Nicotine causes extreme peristalsis and intestinal spasm and for that reason some people use smoking as a laxative. Nicotine causes blood pressure to go up, while the dermal blood vessels contract so that people who are heavy smokers have a pallid appearance. In that nicotine causes the bile ducts to contract, people with liver or gall bladder trouble often find that smoking does not agree with them. Smoking affects the nervous system and heavy smoking can cause nervous excitability. People prone to nervousness would be well advised to refrain from smoking. Many smokers find that when they are tired and have a cigarette, they feel less fatigue. This is due to the fact that nicotine obscures the sensations of tiredness, yet it does not really render the person less tired; it merely masks the complete tiredness for awhile. Smoking uses up vitamin C with the result that smokers suffer from a vitamin C deficiency unless they take much larger than normal amounts each day. Vitamin C deficiency renders one much more suspectible to infectious diseases.

At the American Medical Association meeting held in Dallas, Texas in 1959, Dr. Oscar Auerbach presented the results of extensive and exacting research done by himself, Dr. Arthur Purdy Sout (retired professor of Pathology at Columbia University's College of Physicians and Surgeons), and Dr. E. Cuyler Hammond and Lawrence Garfinkel, both of the American Cancer Society. They made microscopic examinations of 19,797 specimens of tissue from human lungs, and found that the anatomical evidence clearly shows that smoking can cause lung cancer. Up until this time there had been some question about the complete validity of past research projects which indicated very strongly that there was a relationship between smoking and lung cancer. With this study, there could be no doubt about the high correlation that exists between lung cancer and smoking. When one smokes, he is taking a calculated risk about the chances of eventually getting lung cancer, in addition to the other harmful effects which smoking may eventually have upon the system.

Alcohol is the most misunderstood of all the so-called stimulants, though it is more aptly described as a depressant. Unlike coffee, tea and tobacco, alcoholic beverages have been in use as long as civilization has been known. They represent one of man's earliest discoveries.

Higher life could not exist without alcohol in that carbohydrates, starch and sugar form alcohol when they decompose. As such, normal alcohol enters the blood stream following each meal. In this manner, it is normal for the blood to have approximately one gram of alcohol circulating through the body at one time. This is normal and necessary, but more than that renders an abnormal situation. In that alcohol enters the blood stream almost directly, the amount in the blood stream at any given time can be determined simply by blood analysis. That is why many people are given a blood test following an automobile accident to determine if they are, or are not, intoxicated, and if so, the degree of inebriation.

Actually alcohol is a narcotic similar to chloroform and ether, but is very much weaker. A narcotic is any substance which has a particular relationship to the fats of the nervous system by penetrating rapidly into the nerve cells and causing a paralyzing influence upon them. But, before a narcotic paralysis, it creates a state of excitation by stimulating the nerve cells. Alcohol exerts a depressing effect upon the brain, especially those areas which control reflexes, observation and attention. The extent to which alcohol will have these effects upon an individual depends upon two factors—his general constitution and tolerance for alcohol, and the amount consumed.

Dr. Roger Williams, head of the Biochemical Institute of the University of Texas, stresses the fact that some people are more susceptible to alcoholism than others due to their heredity. This seems to be accounted for in that they have inborn nutritional demands, which are exceptionally high, making them susceptible to deficiencies that others do not have. It seems then that alcoholism is of a hereditary nature expressing itself through the malfunctioning of the endocrine glands, as these are affected by diet and nutrition. It has been my experience that most alcoholics, who have been under my care for correction of their chemistry, suffered from an underactive posterior pituitary gland. Usually a posterior pituitary gland deficiency is indicated by an unusual desire for either sugar or alcohol, the former may be termed sugarholics while the latter are alcoholics. When their body chemistry has been brought to normal functioning through administering of the proper amount of posterior pituitary gland extract plus other glandular supplements that may be needed in addition to a wholesome, natural diet, the individuals ceased to suffer from alcoholism. In all cases, the symptoms are practically the same, but in that each person is an individual different from anyone else, the glandular supplement must be determined especially for him according to the specific needs of his body.

Alcohol interferes with and inhibits the action of vitamins. When alcohol is in the liver, the liver has trouble manufacturing vitamin A from carotene. Excess alcohol in the system slows the absorption and reaction of vitamin B^1 which explains the nervous symptoms common to acute alcoholism. Furthermore it seems that too much alcohol in the system interferes with the absorption of vitamins B^2, C and K. Pellagra if often a serious consequence of chronic alcoholism, as well as cirrhosis of the liver, neuritis, mental disturbances and premature senility. Evidence indicates that alcohol may be toxic to the reproductive cells of the body and thus may affect the hereditary processes.

Taken in strict moderation, alcohol affects the blood sugar level and calcium-phosphorus levels much less than coffee and sugar, but when consumed in excessive amounts, it upsets body chemistry and has a detrimental effect upon the glands. The use of excessive alcohol has the same disastrous consequences as the eating of sugar and white flour. Alcohol has a caloric value, but its value is like the empty calories of sugar and white flour; they all affect the glands and hence body metabolism by reducing hunger. Alcohol, sugar, coffee, white flour and tea all hinder the digestion of vital foods that are rich in constructive and protective nutrients, which the body must have to maintain normal health.

Alcoholism, as such, seems to be both a hereditary and dietary problem. Through the body chemistry approach to sound health, alcoholism may often be cured. This involves endocrine glandular supplementation as needed by the given individual and a good, wholesome diet that excludes those processed and unnatural foods so characteristic of the modern way of life.

VI.   Degenerative Diseases

Now that infant mortality and infectious diseases have been brought under control and largely conquered, it is the degenerative diseases that are taking so many lives and young lives at that. Most of us assume that we are much better off than our parents and grandparents of 1900 due to the widely publicized lengthening of the life span in America. We think that we will live to reach 65 or 75 and perhaps more. The life expectancy of 1900 was 50 and that of 1960 was 70, but that does not mean that one has a particularly greater chance of living to be 70. Due to this type of publicity, many people erroneously conclude that they have a better chance of reaching 75 than did their parents. Such an assumption is not justified as the facts will bear out. What these statistics mean is that through cutting infant mortality to a minimum and by controlling infectious diseases, more people are permitted to live to adulthood. You can see that when you mathematically average the death of infants and children with that of the death of adults, it will give you a smaller total figure. In that most people born in the United States reach maturity today, means that they have grown up only to become afflicted with degenerative diseases. Actually, the life expectancy of a man of 60 today is only a year and a half longer than that of a man of 60 in 1900. That does not represent much of an increase, and since few people die in childhood, the mathematical picture makes it look as if life expectancy has greatly increased. Even with the control of infectious diseases by our antibiotic drugs, a middle aged man of today has very little more chance of reaching 75 than did the middle aged man in 1900 when so many people died of flu, pneumonia and numerous other infectious diseases. In fact, the number of people dying in the middle age bracket from chronic degenerative diseases, such as heart attacks, circulatory diseases, cancer and many others, is on the increase to such an extent that the mathematical life expectancy is beginning to go down.

As infectious diseases have been largely conquered or controlled, degenerative diseases are on the galloping increase. Why is this? The answer lies in the malfunctioning of body chemistry brought about by hereditary factors and particularly by an inadequate and unhealthy diet that puts undue stress and strain upon the endocrine glands, with the inevitable result that they function inefficiently. Eventually degenerative diseases of one type or another set in. Dr. Tom D. Spies, the internationally noted medical nutritionist, noted that if the human body is kept in proper chemical balance, it would grow old with little mental and physical deterioration.

Dr. Paul C. Aebersold of the Isotopes Division of the Atomic Energy Commission, through his research by using radioactive isotopes, proved that about 98 per cent of the cells of the body are replaced each year through the air, food and drink we take into our bodies. When a person realizes what this means it points up the extreme importance of proper diet, namely one which furnished him with all the various substances he needs and omits those substances which are harmful to the body. Every day that he obeys the natural laws of nutrition, he is making his body over to some degree in a more healthful manner.

Autopsies were performed upon 300 soldiers who were killed in action in the Korean War and it was startling to discover that 77.3 per cent of them had heart disease. These soldiers fell in the age group of the late teens and early twenties for the most part with an average age of 22. Already at that young age, they were suffering from degenerative disease, yet this did not manifest itself openly. Why were so many young men suffering from such a degenerative disease? Dr. Pauline Berry Mack, the outstanding and well-known nutritional authority, probably has the answer for us.

She made a study of 2,536 girls and boys falling between the ages of 13 and 20. These young people would be considered to have an excellent diet in that they ate what is generally considered to provide good nutrition and it did represent the typical American diet. Dr. Mack found that about three-fourths of these young people were not eating enough of the energy making foods necessary to keep the body machinery working efficiently; they did not eat enough protein, and forty-eight per cent of them suffered from what she termed "nutritional nerves"—biting of the finger nails, restlessness, and twitching of the face. Most all of these 2,536 boys and girls had marked vitamin deficiencies. She concluded that children needed to be fed a good, sound diet and noted that a well-balanced, natural, wholesome diet usually costs less than a poor diet consisting of cake, milk shakes and all the other processed foods that make up the greater part of the modern American diet.

In the United States there are eleven million people suffering from crippling arthritis. It is our country's most widespread chronic disease. There are a number of different types of arthritis. Rheumatoid arthritis is a generalized disease of the entire body that produces an inflammation of the joints; osteo-arthritis attacks the bone and cartilege in the joints; in gout a chalky substance is deposited especially in the joint tissues of the hands and feet; with cataracts a deposit is put over the eye; while with pyorrhea, that part of the jaw bone which supports the teeth dissolves, causing inflammation of the gums which eventually necessitates removal of the teeth.

Arthritis generally is defined as inflammation of a joint. Pericementitis is also inflammation of a joint—the tooth joint—and is the forerunner of pyorrhea. The chief difference between pyorrhea and arthritis is that pyorrhea can be treated locally without great difficulty. Soothing lotions can be applied directly to the inflamed areas and irritating deposits can be readily removed by instrumentation which gives relief but no real cure.

Inflamed joints, covered by soft tissue, are not readily accessible to medication and instrumentation. The treatment must of necessity be nearly all systemic. Since pericementitis and arthritis are but symptoms of the same disease, systemic treatment is equally applicable to them. From the dental standpoint, while the disease may be alleviated by local treatment without treatment designed to correct the disease from a basic standpoint, nothing is done to prevent its recurrence either at the tooth joint or some other joint. Assuming that arthritis encompasses pyorrhea, pericementitis and gingivitis and are diseases of disturbed metabolism directly influenced by calcium-phosphorus levels of the blood, we would find these levels out of balance where the disease occurs and balance should bring relief from its symptoms. This is the case.

The onset of the disease is usually marked by pain and tenderness. It may or may not be accompanied by swelling. In this acute stage, we have repeatedly found that the calcium level of the blood is low and the phosphorus level is high. If bony structures are affected, there is a withdrawal of calcium, and if this stage lasts long enough, a dissolving process is evidenced by means of the X ray. This stage or type of arthritis is called the "dissolving stage." Since movement of the affected parts elicits increased pain and increases the inflammatory process, rest is essential for the parts affected.

The initial process is usually not of long duration. In a few weeks the inflammation usually subsides and the patient may not have another attack for years and possibly forever. The chances are, however, that unless the cause is eliminated, the attacks will recur with ever increasing frequency.

The periods between acute attacks, at first, are often symptomless, except for slight pain with unusual movement or a slight, scarcely noticeable stiffness. But with increased frequency of acute attacks, discomfort of the in-between periods is more marked. At these times, we find the calcium levels high and the phosphorus levels low. X rays show that there is a tendency of the uncombined calcium to deposit in the etched areas resulting from the previous acute stage. For this reason, it is called the "depositing stage."

The dissolving or acute stage may in a small proportion of cases persist for long periods of time with very little of the depositing stage, or the depositing stage may persist with no history of the acute stage. Both types of cases are illustrated by two elderly sisters, cripples, whose time was spent either in bed, or in wheelchairs. One had the dissolving type of arthritis, or what might be called the prolonged acute stage, to the degree that the bones of the fingers and toes had completely disappeared. The other sister had the depositing form of arthritis or arthritis deformans. Her hands and feet were gnarled and club-like. Most of her joints were permanently ankylosed. This sister later had her leg amputated because of gangrene. The arteries had become so occluded with calcium that it was practically a bloodless operation. Both cases resulted from disturbed body chemistry.

The ordinary case of arthritis is characterized by alternating high and low levels of phosphorus in which the acute or dissolving stage rarely lasts more than six weeks, and the chronic or depositing stage is the usual stage in which the individual lives. The patient often thinks that he is over his arthritis in this later stage, and that his stiffness is but the result of the acute stage.

Although faulty body chemistry is the cause of arthritis, there are a number of causes for this faulty body chemistry. Hence treatment to cure the disease depends upon recognition of the factor or factors responsible. Mental conditions may so affect the body chemistry that there is a wide fluctuation of calcium and phosphorus levels. During times of depression, many business men develop aches and pains from worry that later disappear with the return of more normal business conditions.

Mechanical conditions can produce defective chemistry

of a part by interference with normal circulation, as witness Pemberton's experiment in tying off part of the blood supply in a dog's leg, which resulted in arthritic deposits. Arthritis in the shoulder may come from a sleeping posture producing interference with circulation.

Infection usually affects the body chemistry. When infection is the cause, its removal usually clears up the arthritis. Infection, however, is but one factor which may affect body chemistry. The greatest mistake in the treatment of arthritis has been the supposition that there must always be infection at the root of the disease. Thousands of mouths have been wrecked by the needless extraction of teeth, to say nothing of the removal of tonsils, gall bladders, appendices, and whatnot, all to no avail. Even these measures have generally given some temporary relief in chronic forms of arthritis, for the healing process following the operation serves to raise the phosphorus level, often sufficiently so that the patient feels sure for awhile that the cause of his trouble has been found and removed. Disillusionment comes later and the search for infection continues. I believe this phenomenon of apparent relief after an operation has misled many of the profession to the belief that arthritis is always due to infection.

When infection is the cause of arthritis, we have found the most usual source to be tonsil tags or stumps, pyorrhea and devitalized teeth which are second in order, and kidney infection, the third. The differential blood picture usually will have a high white count, a high stab count, and a high sedimentation rate when infection exists. An attempt is made to approximately locate the source of the infection and to send the patient to the specialist needed.

X rays are of prime necessity in ruling on the health of the teeth and surrounding structures. Pressure on the jugular vein according to the technic of Dr. Otto Meyer of New York will determine inflammation to be present or absent in this vein. If present, the patient will wince at slight pressure. This according to Dr. Meyer indicates the presence of infection somewhere in the vicinity of the jugular vein. This most often is in the tonsilar region. He reports that about 98 per cent of the tonsils removed in the past were done incompletely. The stumps which remain then become a continuing source of infection as they can no longer drain into the throat as intended because of the scar tissue covering them.

When there is no pain upon pressure, the patient usually has his tonsils intact. From my experience in this regard in the last few years, I would surmise that more tonsillectomies have been performed than were needed. Microscopic analysis of the urine will usually indicate if there is any infection of kidneys, bladder or other sections of the urinary tract.

The cause of arthritis may be in the diet; not in meats that are red, as once was thought, but in an inadequate diet; a diet deficient in one or more of the essentials needed by the body. Dr. Charles A. Brusch and Dr. Edward T. Johnson, both outstanding medical physicians, reported in the July 1959 issue of *The Journal of the National Medical Association* that diet produced significantly clinical improvements in arthritis and rheumatism. They further noted an improvement in the blood. The diet that they prescribe is very similar to the one I have been using for years, the so-called basic or Page Diet which eliminates refined carbohydrates—sugar, soft drinks, coffee, cake, candy, milk, hydrogenated fats, ice cream and any foods made with sugar. Dr. Brusch and Dr. Johnson also found that on the specific diet they had their patients follow, that cholesterol levels also dropped or could be controlled, while blood sugar levels returned to normal or near normal. Even one diabetic patient no longer needed to take insulin and blood pressure levels came to nearer normal levels. In my clinical practice, it has been found that the diets of arthritics are preponderantly carbohydrate and deficient in the trace minerals. Usually a deficiency of the B vitamins is found if the diet consists in any part of refined carbohydrates, for even a good diet is not apt to have too much of the B vitamins for optimal health. In this respect, refined carbohydrates, such as sugar, displace by the number of calories they contain an equal number of calories of life-containing foods.

In a series of several hundred arthritics, nearly all consumed large quantities of sugar. Sugar disturbs calcium-phosphorus balance more than any single factor. It disturbs it in the direction of higher calcium and lower phosphorus. When the effect of the sugar has worn off, there is a rebound in the opposite direction; for action equals reaction.

Nutritional treatment, therefore, consists of a diet which contains all of the essentials the body needs, and does not contain substances which the body is unequipped to handle efficiently. The latter things are principally white flour, sugar, coffee, hydrogenated fat, milk, and alcohol. The modified diabetic diet is the ideal diet for the arthritic, as well as for nearly everyone else. It is the biologic diet.

Menopausal arthritis is due to disturbed glandular function, which is increased at the time of menopause. The disturbance in body chemistry may not have been severe enough prior to the time of menopause to create any distressing symptoms. It might be noted at this time that menopause is but a normal process in people whose body chemistry is normal, but if the body chemistry is abnormal, the period then becomes one of physical and mental stress. Treatment of arthritis of this origin is chiefly endocrine and nutritional.

Symptomatic treatment for the immediate relief of pain consists of the use of endocrine products because it is wisest to follow the rules of nature and use those products that nature uses to maintain equilibrium of body chemistry. A little augmentation of the body's own endocrine products often serves the body well and in a way most acceptable to the body.

Sugar raises the calcium level and lowers the phosphorus level. Honey will do the same but since honey contains valuable food ingredients in addition to sugar, it can be used in strict moderation. A tablespoon or more at each meal to relieve the pain in acute arthritis is of great benefit, for if the phosphorus level is dropped to forty per cent of the calcium level, the inflammation will usually disappear with a few hours.

The response to insulin therapy in these acute cases is often spectacular, but these measures must be stopped as soon as this stage subsides. After the acute stage is over, the treatment is largely nutritional. This may be augmented by endocrine therapy. The blood should be checked at frequent intervals to keep track of the proportion of phosphorus to calcium. All glandular substances are cumulative in action and the phosphorus level may rise past the 40 per cent mark and cause a return of the acute symptoms.

Experimentally, the author has done this several times and more than once unintentionally. Discontinuance of the extract for a few days before resuming at a lessened amount will suffice to terminate the acute symptoms.

The object of nutritional treatment is to correct endocrine function. Endocrine substitution or augmentation is at best a crude method of furnishing the desired hormones. It is impossible to supply the products at the natural rate of glandular secretion, or to know exactly just what secretions need augmentation. It is difficult to judge how much substance should be given even with the calcium-phosphorus levels as a guide. Without them it had been mostly pure guess.

Allergy is another cause of rheumatic pain. This is not always reflected in the calcium-phosphorus levels. The author knows of two cases where lumbago was caused by the drinking of coffee. Coffee with the caffeine removed did not have this effect.

It is to be emphasized, however, that the control of arthritis lies only in the reversal of the process which depleted the efficiency of the body chemistry. A new name for the many centuries old diet of our fathers is the "biologic diet." It is composed of essentially the same materials, though possibly in different form, as was the food of our ancestors. It produced strong sturdy people, and is just as well fitted for us now as it was for them. Our modern civilized diets differ from the biologic diet principally by the introduction of refined foods. With the elimination of these refined foods, the instincts which guided our ancestors in the selection of food once more take charge. Without fail, our instincts guide us to the biologic diet providing it is available. As demonstrated by Dr. Richter of John Hopkins University, the lack of common sense on the part of mankind in the control of foods has produced the digestive chaos which calls for an army of nutritional experts. The perfection of nutritional science hands this control back to nature again. We must remember that although our environment has changed, the bodies in which we live are the same as they were a thousand years ago, so far as chemical function is concerned.

On the biologic diet along with endocrine supplement, the arthritic may expect to gradually increase the efficiency of his body chemistry and, as he does so, the arthritis will gradually disappear. It is understood, of course, that the scars, so-to-speak, of the arthritis may persist for a long time, if not forever. There is also a great difference in the ability of different people to respond to nutritional treatment. This does not depend so much on the age of the individual as it does on the duration of the nutritional inadequacy. This is calculated in generations rather than years. If the patient's immediate ancestors were from Europe, where nutritional conditions on the whole have been better than in the United States, the patient's response is usually prompt. Where the patient's immediate ancestors were Americans, the response is less prompt, and if several generations of Americans precede the patient, the response is apt to be slow.

A case will illustrate:

A young man of twenty-seven came with a multiplicity of ills. He had badly inflamed gums, a devitalized tooth, arthritis of the hands and feet and psoriasis.

The psoriasis, a skin disease, diagnosed by an eminent dermatologist, had resisted treatment for fourteen years. It occurred in large patches over the body and through the hair. At times, the thick scales dropped off in showers, at other times the exudation penetrated his clothes. Because of the arthritis, this young missionary had been sent back from Alaska and physicians had told him that he could never return to such a severe climate. His church had given him a year's leave of absence to improve his health, as his badly swollen and painful hands and feet interfered with his work. The devitalized tooth was extracted and local treatment given for the inflamed condition of the gums.

It was believed that systemic treatment to correct the gum conditions would also have an effect on the other symptoms of disorder. The patient was put on the Page Diet and given glandular treatment as indicated by his endocrinagraph and as verified by blood analysis. Gradually, the patient was taught to watch the color of his gums. If bright red and inflamed, he was to come for an insulin injection. If not, he was to take only posterior pituitary gland extract in amounts which he learned to regulate according to the condition of his hands. If pain occurred, he could take as high as one and one-half tenth grains of posterior pituitary tablets; if no pain, he was to take as little as was necessary to maintain that state. Within a few weeks, he learned that he could control the arthritis pain through this means if he did not expose the weakened joints to undue exercise or cold. Swelling was slower to respond to this treatment than the pain, but that, too, finally disappeared. Along with this, began a gradual disappearance of the psoriasis. First, the inner portions of the patches faded, then the stubborn outer rings faded out and finally, with exposure to sun and salt water, the patches over his entire body disappeared, leaving only faint scars. The patient, happy as could be, went to the dermatologist to show him what had happened under systemic treatment where local treatment had failed.

This patient proved a valuable source of information as to the diet of the primitive Eskimo. He fully corroborates Doctors Price and Waugh and states that the Eskimo uses seal or other animal fat for the purpose for which he used candy—namely, to give warmth and quick energy. Besides containing heat units in the proportion of nine to four as compared to candy, natural fat furnishes normal heat and energy as intended by nature; whereas sugars do so by upsetting the body's chemistry.

Another case of arthritis was of a woman fifty-two years of age, of English ancestry on one side and Holland-French on the other. She was the typical American of long-headed Nordic ancestry. She lived in Detroit; her parents before her had lived in Wisconsin and Michigan.

Her diet was just about typical of the American diet of people of her station in life. She ate meat, eggs, fish (mostly fresh-water), two slices of whole wheat bread daily. She had cereal of some kind at breakfast and ate all kinds of vegetables, both raw and cooked, as well as orange or tomato juice at least once per day, but she drank six cups of coffee daily, in each of which she used one teaspoon of sugar. That, with one teasponful for her cereal, made seven. Besides this, she ate candy, cake, cookies and canned fruit, all of which contain large quantities of refined sugar. She had begun to lose her pep in the last few years, and so had become accustomed to taking two cocktails and a highball each day. She also smoked about a package of cigarettes daily.

After two months on the Page Diet her calcium level began to rise and in three months the calcium and phosphorus levels were once more in balance. All symptoms of arthritis disappeared. She was particularly pleased to report that she had danced all evening at a party—something she had been unable to do for some time.

This case had a favorable outcome in other respects. It showed how behavior often reflects the state of the body chemistry. She had used alcoholic drinks regularly only for the last two years. She explained that she felt better when taking them and decided that since she was a grandmother now, she had a right to do as she pleased, if it made her more comfortable.

It is interesting to note that after this woman's body

chemistry became more efficient, she ceased to feel the need for sugar, coffee and alcoholic drinks daily. She also ceased to be a smoker.

A man of forty-five suffering from acute arthritis in his hands came to our attention. His history was interesting and the outcome of treatment amazing. As a new employee he learned about the harmful effects of sugar upon body chemistry and voluntarily ceased its use. Under ordinary circumstances this would have been beneficial but in his case it was disastrous. For a number of years this man had been drinking a pint of liquor daily and occasionally went on a week's binge as well. He had completely given up liquor two months previous to our acquaintance with him. By ceasing both sugar and alcohol, he had knocked the props out from under his faulty body chemistry. Unwittingly, he had used excessive amounts of sugar and alcohol to maintain a calcium level consistent with the high phosphorus level produced by his faulty body chemistry.

The too-sudden drop in the man's calcium level made him acutely ill. The inflammation of his gums increased, he had a high temperature, rapid pulse, raised blood pressure, severe pains in his hands and was in a state of delirium for some days. It was not until he was given posterior pituitary tablets that the inflammation of his gums and hands decreased. By regular blood tests, daily checks of his temperature, specific gravity of his urine, and the color of his gums, the dosage of posterior pituitary was increased to two and one-half tenths of a grain per day. The swelling and pain in his hands disappeared, the blood calcium-phosphorus approached normal and his desire for sweets and alcohol was as if it had never been. The daily intake of posterior pituitary gland extract was gradually reduced as the blood tests indicated basic improvement of the functioning of this patient's body chemistry.

During seven years the amount of posterior pituitary substance has been reduced gradually, so that now he is taking 3/400 of a grain daily. We take this to mean that his own posterior pituitary gland has almost regained normal function. If you figure it out, you will find that the amount has been reduced to 1/33 of the original dose. He has thus established and maintained balanced body chemistry with the result that he now enjoys good health.

We have had many cases similar to this one, and from our experience with these alcoholics and with hundreds of sugar addicts, we know that these people are really very sick. They are usually deficient in posterior pituitary secretion and as a result have too little calcium and too much phosphorus in the blood. This condition produces a state of nervous irritation, which is relieved by alcohol raising the calcium level of the blood and lowering the phosphorus level at the same time.

Another typical arthritic case is that of Mr. C., a road contractor of fifty-five, weight 204 pounds and height of six feet.

He was always tired, had frequent colds, and did not like cold weather. He ate no sugar but did eat pie, canned fruit, and white bread. Blood tests showed that he had a high calcium level. He was treated with thyroid 3/10 of a grain per day for two weeks, 2/10 of a grain daily for two weeks and 1/10 of a grain daily for four months and then endocrine treatment ceased. In the meantime, we took him off sugar and foods containing sugar. Since he was a blue-eyed Swede we knew that his dietary requirements should include a high amount of trace minerals. As his calcium level was reduced towards normal, there was a gradual lessening of deposits. And so long as he continues to be in chemical balance, he will be free of arthritis. Incidentally, his blood pressure also returned to normal.

A lady of fifty-three years of age, who had been suffering from crippling arthritis since 1948, came to us seeking a solution to her difficulties.

For some years she had been treated by specialists and had taken cortisone and other drugs, all of which gave some temporary relief for a short period of time and then her condition seemed to become worse. It has been well established that cortisone, ACTH, gold salts, and the like often give temporary relief to arthritic sufferers. But in the long run, continued use of them usually renders the patient in a worse condition than when he began taking them. This lady was of English-German ancestry. Arthritis had terribly deformed both the hands, fingers, and toes, and she could hardly walk. Her anthropometric graph indicated that she was exceptionally gynic while everything else approached normal. Her blood sugar was on the low side. She was put on the Page Diet which eliminates all sugar and sugar products, coffee, milk, white flour and refined grains, and hydrogenated fats. Through blood analysis the minute dosage of testosterone suitable to her special needs was determined. Within a very short time she made remarkable improvement and within a year she had regained full movement of her legs and partial movement of her fingers. The excruciating pain had disappeared and she was able to move around with ease, even to climb stairs. Although the complete crippling features caused by the arthritis could not be entirely undone, further progress of the disease was stopped and the tide was turned as is evidenced by the free movement which returned to her previously stiff fingers and joints.

A young college student of nineteen, suffering from symptoms of arthritis, was referred to us. He was a fine looking gentleman of Irish-Scotch extraction and seemingly in excellent health except for excess weight. However on close examination one could notice knots on the joints of his stiff fingers. He often suffered from dull, agonizing pain in both hands and knees. His family history consisted of many cases of diabetes. He was on the regular American diet except for consuming more coffee than usual in that he had a part-time job working at night. His endocrinograph was good except for indicating an overactive posterior pituitary gland function. Blood analysis showed that he had a very high blood sugar which indicated a condition of pre-diabetes while his cholesterol level was slightly high. He was put on the Page Diet and given three units of insulin per day. Within two weeks time he began to feel better and his blood sugar and cholesterol level came to normal. Within four months the knots and stiffness of his fingers had disappeared, all symptoms of arthritis went away, and he had lost his thirty pounds of overweight. At this time the insulin was stopped and he was kept on the Page Diet alone. It seemed that, given a chance, his body and glands had recuperated and he needed no further glandular supplementation. This often happens and is the rule with young people. This boy has had no further difficulties. He states that he will stay on the Page Diet because he knows how important it is. He is a wise chap, but it took a little pain and some worrying to snap him out of his lethargy. Most people are willing to try anything when they get "desperate" or have pain. It would be so much simpler if we would but learn to take care of our bodies properly and thus prevent many of these things happening in the first place. But being only human, we usually do not think that far ahead, yet the answer is within the reach of everyone.

In my clinical experience with cataracts, which are a type of depositional arthritis of the eyes obstructing vision, if the excess calcium can be eliminated and sound body chemistry established, the results are good. This method is very satisfactory in incipient cataracts, but if the cataracts get dense enough to block off vision completely, there is little chance for reversal of these deposits. A good analogy is as follows: When a river is moving it often piles up sand at a turn and thus makes a sand bar. In time, the river may slightly change course, and if the sand bar has not become solidified and firmly set, the swift movement of the current will wear it down and carry the sand bar away. However, if it has become firmly set and has dense vegetation growing on it, it will stand firm and remain permanently. This is the case with cataracts. If they have not become firmly set, they may be reabsorbed into the system with the establishment of good body chemistry.

Miss A. was a most unusual case, for although only eighteen, she had cataracts. Like her immediate ancestors she was a Southerner of Irish stock. Her vision was reduced to 10 per cent of normal. She had a good position as secretary and assistant to a dentist but, naturally, her fear of losing her eyesight was coupled with the fear of losing her job. No one knew how serious her handicap was because she always deciphered her notes when alone by the aid of a reading glass. She had unusually large, well curved breasts. She had plenty of pep and was a very attractive young lady. Excesses in her diet were found in beer, soft drinks, and sugar. She was a chain smoker, using nicotine to quiet her jittery nerves.

Miss A's. higher than normal blood pressure, inordinate pep and the distribution of weight above the waist led to a diagnosis necessitating insulin injections regularly. Her diet was corrected. The use of cigarettes was gradually lessened. Within three months her 10 per cent vision had increased to 50 per cent but after that we were baffled as she ceased to make any further progress. It was decided to re-study the case. Thyroid and vitamin B were given, and posterior pituitary gland extract. Improvement began again.

After about a year and a half of the correct endocrine treatment, plus strict adherence to the Page Diet, Miss A. was well. There were no signs of cataracts and there has been no return of symptoms since that time. But there were other changes which occurred besides the return of vision. She attained a more normal weight by losing nine pounds, her breasts were no longer so large and she was in excellent health.

A gentleman of seventy, who was blind in one eye due to an injury sustained in childhood, began to have symptoms of cataract in his eye of vision. His endocrinograph indicated that he was overactive in the production of male hormones and that the function of the anterior pituitary gland was not working properly. He was put on the Page Diet and given two 1/1200 tablets of estrogen per day along with three units of insulin and one unit of adrenal cortex solution. To the complete astonishment of everyone he regained full sight of his blind eye and then, as expected, all symptoms of the cataract in his good eye disappeared. This gentleman is now in his 80's and has had no further difficulty with his eyes nor with his condition of health in general.

The greatest killer of all the prevalent degenerative diseases are the heart and circulatory diseases which strike thousands upon thousands in their early forties and fifties. It is interesting to note, according to the American Heart Association, that the death rate from cardiovascular diseases is one-third higher among males than females and that between the ages of 35 to 64 the death rate among men from diseases of the heart and blood vessels is on the increase at an alarming rate. It has been noted by many medical researchers that the victims of heart and circulatory diseases are usually the so-called "go-getters" who are constantly driving themselves. In 1959 Dr. Meyer Friedman told the American Heart Association in Philadelphia that a link connecting a person's behavior in a stressful occupation, through hormone channels secreted by the endocrine glands, was related to the vital arteries that supply the heart.. The medical research of Dr. William Sheldon of Columbia University Medical School has also shown a relationship or correlation between the susceptibility to developing heart and circulatory degenerative diseases and body type. All of this corresponds very significantly with the research and clinical findings of Dr. Page and his associates. It is within the realm of body chemistry that the answer to the causes and means of preventing degenerative diseases of this type are to be found. If the answer is within body chemistry, it is natural to ask why such findings have not spread like wildfire. The answer is the same as with Louis Pasteur and his great discoveries which took well over half a century to become accepted. The average mind, even the intelligent mind, hesitates to accept something from an unexpected source. Man does not often accept new and revolutionary ideas immediately—they must penetrate slowly as was the case with Copernicus, Galileo, and Pasteur. Nevertheless, in time, once the basic premise for tracking down this enemy of man is agreed upon, acceptance of the findings by a dentist will be welcomed.

Heart disease is a degenerative process due to a breakdown within the host, precipitated in some cases by the trigger mechanism of infectious disease but basically due to weakness within the host itself. Degenerative disease has always been the field of the dentist. The dentist has treated body ills from the beginning as has the medical doctor. Only the dentist has been a specialist from the beginning, a specialist in degenerative processes in one part of the body, whereas until recent date the medical doctor has treated the whole body with emphasis upon epidemic and infectious diseases. Between these two professions has lain a no man's land. For the benefit of patients, for the establishment of a basic attack upon degenerative ills wherever they may occur in the body, this gap, this no man's land, must be closed. This will not require domination by the medical profession or the dental profession, but collective effort based on mutual respect by each for the work of the other.

To answer why more males are coronary victims, where the weakening factor in the patient is to be found, and how to recognize it, should indicate the proper course for both prevention and correction. Let us follow this out one step at a time.

Why are more males coronary victims? What is the basic difference between maleness and femaleness? It is the degree of male hormones or female hormones of each as compared to the other—the degree to which each mechanism is more anabolic or catabolic in its function. In everyday parlance, anabolic means to build up and catabolic to wear down. Male hormones mean more catabolic factors than anabolic, the organism tends to wear itself down as opposed to female hormones which tend to build up. The anabolic organism tends to withstand more strain than the catabolic. The increased longevity of women over men is a case in point. The average life of women used to be three years greater than that of man, but it has now increased to an average life expectancy for women of six years more than that of her male counterpart. During the same period of time in which the longevity of women as compared to men has increased, the number of deaths from coronary ills has also increased.

Studies of body chemistry should indicate the predominance of either anabolic or catabolic factors and, therefore, should show a relationship to longevity. The Page Foundation tested a group of men and women from 75 to 94 years of age (Members of the Three-Quarter Century Club of St. Petersburg) for bodily efficiency. The tests were revealing for two reasons: (1) all those tested showed a higher level of bodily efficiency than is found in the average individual; (2) among the men there was a lower level of male hormone production than is found in the average male.

Seemingly we have two factors augmenting each other; (1) females live longer than males, (2) those males who are long-lived have less male hormones than the average male. Statistics clearly prove that the majority of coronary victims are short-lived. How do coronary cases register in a test for maleness? (a) Tests of their body efficiency indicate a greater activity of the catabolic glands than found in the average, and (b) a greater amount of male hormones than found in the average male. Our conclusion, therefore, is that males are more often victims of coronary ills because of their excessive production of male hormones.

The answer to the second question, where in the victim is the weakening factor or factors to be found, was implied in the discussion of "Why?": According to tests for the degree of body efficiency of the patient, the catabolic glands are more overactive in heart cases, and the glands controlling maleness are more active than in the average male. The observation that women with a history of coronary ills show a greater degree of activity of the catabolic glands, and more male factors than the average woman, is further indication that this line of reasoning is at least headed in the right direction. Furthermore, medical men themselves are approaching this point of view in their research into the relationship of estrogen (female hormone) to the control of coronary ills. For example medical research, carried out by investigators at the University of Southern California School of Medicine, reports that by administering a small amount of estrogen to middle-aged patients they are rendered less susceptible to heart attacks. Dr. Jessie Marmorston took 174 women, many past 70, who had had one or more heart attacks and divided them into two equal groups. One-half of them received a small daily dose of estrogen while the other half received none. After three years, more than twice as many in the group who had not received estrogen had died from new heart attacks or their disease had become steadily worse. Dr. Oliver Kuzma, who is working with Dr. Marmorston, had about the same to report from a group of 109 men who were given a little larger, but non-feminizing dose of estrogen than the women had received. Also, Dr. Kuzma found that in most cases the levels of cholesterol and additional fat fractions circulating in the blood of heart attack victims returned closer to normal when a small amount of estrogen was given.

Estrogen is the female sex hormone which is secreted by both males and females, but women, quite naturally, produce more than man. It is the so-called feminizing hormone, but it actually has many vital qualities. Each sex must have this vital hormone in the proper proportions in order to have a healthy functioning body. It seems that this hormone is important in preventing heart diseases, because from the early teens to the early fifties women suffer only a negligible amount of heart attacks; but after menopause women progressively secrete less estrogen until around the age of seventy-five, at which age the female then becomes very susceptible to heart attacks so report Dr. Kuzma and Dr. Marmorston.

The body chemistry approach to good health, as developed and expounded by the author, has long recognized the importance of estrogen and the other hormones in establishing normal health which will enable one to live the full life span of his natural endowed heredity. However, in my clinical practice I long ago realized that estrogen should not be given to everyone who is in or past middle age, but should be administered only to those who actually need it, and this very often includes the young. The Page anthropometric graph usually tells the story; that is, it will show whether your bodily inheritance predestines you to have too much estrogen, too little, or just the right amount. This is termed the andro-gynic balance. To give estrogen to a person who already has too much is just making a bad situation worse; likewise, to give too much to one who does not have enough will only complicate his ailment—in fact, the patient just goes from bad to worse. But when just the right amount is given along with the basic diet and other endocrines are needed, if any, good response is to be expected. After all, good body chemistry merely means establishing the proper hormone balance for the given individual and then keeping his body chemistry efficient through taking the endocrine supplement in the proper dosage (which is determined by the graph and blood analysis), eating only a proper natural diet and using natural vitamins if recommended.

In dealing with people, no two of whom are identical, each must be dealt with as an individual and, as such, one cannot prescribe that everyone suffering from a specific degenerative disease (and heart attacks fall into that category) should receive the same amount of the same hormone or even the same treatment. The dosage that is just right for one person may be undesirable for another, but when used in the proper amount the results are as desired. Hormones keep our body functioning properly, but to have too many, or to take too many makes for an unhealty body just as too little does. The body chemistry approach is to establish what is need for each individual for his specific needs. In other words, the body chemistry approach to good health treats the whole person as an individual, not just the disease. When good body chemistry has been established, and is maintained, there should be no degenerative disease; as with chemical efficiency each individual should then be expected to live the whole life span with which he was endowed by God and nature. So it is evident from our point of view that the medical profession still has much to learn concerning dosage before it achieves the degree of success possible for correcting coronary ills through this approach. Before the medical profession can use the same means of prevention, they must learn how to recognize candidates for coronary ills in advance of an attack. This latter can be done by measuring the body efficiency of an individual and noting which glands or endocrines (the controllers of body efficiency) are overactive.

Our observation leads us to believe that 97 per cent of coronary ills are basically due to overactivity of the thyroid gland and/or the anterior pituitary, plus greater andricity (too much male hormone—testosterone) for the individual (male or female) than is normal. Correction and prevention, therefore, should obviously be directed to inhibition of the overactivity of the thyroid and/or the anterior pituitary with re-balancing of the androgenic (male or female) factors. Since the body produces its own thyroid and anterior pituitary substances, treatment should be based on a plan of supplementation of the opposing glands, not substitution. The body's own production of these materials in a twenty-four hour period is minimal, so supplementation would be fractional; otherwise one type of imbalance will have been substituted for another type of imbalance. Health requires true balance.

Now you have the answer, at least from our point of view, as to the why, where and how of coronary ills. From this can be deduced the method of approach for correction and prevention. That these deductions are not all theory, but have been tried and proven effective, can be shown by case histories, in our office and the offices of our associates, of individuals with inefficient chemistry complicated by coronary ills. As time goes on, let us hope that the barriers between dental doctors and medical doctors can be broken down, so that knowledge may pass freely between them to the advantage of the public and an increase in the health level of the nation.

More and more medical research is throwing light upon the causes of degenerative diseases, all of which points to body chemistry. In October 1959 at a program of the Newspaper Food Conference, Dr. Laurence W. Kinsell, director of the Institute for Metabolic Research at Highland-Alameda County Hospital, Oakland, California, reported the results of research and clinical studies in which it was evidenced that hardening of the arteries, or atherosclerosis, a degenerative disease responsible for heart attacks and strokes, is largely due to a faulty diet and can be largely averted through a proper diet. Dr. Kinsell cited evidence which indicates that hardening of the arteries is not an unavoidable aspect of growing old. He pointed out that heredity and stress are also important factors in leading to atherosclerosis, but that diet is the part of greatest interest in that it is the aspect in which the most can be easily accomplished. Dr. Endel Kask reported in the October 1959 edition of *Angiology, The Journal of Vascular Disease,* that the crucial understanding of heart diseases and especially arteriosclerosis diseases is to be found in the working of hormones and enzymes secreted by the endocrine glands. Diet of course plays a part, in that diet has a significant effect upon the glands, but heredity gives one the glands he will go through life with. If they are not perfect to begin with, then it is necessary to take glandular supplementation to bring about a balance of body chemistry. It is the hormones and enzymes which control the metabolism of lipids which are so important in the development of arteriosclerotic diseases.

Another crucial problem with reference to heart and circulatory diseases is that of blood pressure. High blood pressure, or hypertension, is a degenerative disease that affects approximately ten million people in the United States. At the New York Heart Association conference held in January, 1960, Specialist George A. Perera, M.D. pointed out a number of facts concerning high blood pressure that correlate with the clinical findings of The Page Clinic over the past thirty years. High blood pressure sufferers have many characteristics in common and eventually develop organic complaints that shorten their life expectancy by as much as twenty years. Heredity is a very important factor in high blood pressure. If either of one's parents had it, usually at least one, and perhaps more, of the children will be afflicted. If both parents have had high blood pressure, then most, and maybe all, of the children will suffer from hypertension. Neither personality, stress nor diet causes hypertension, though they may trigger it off, and diet, in the manner in which it affects the glands, plays an important part. To understand high blood pressure requires an understanding of body chemistry, and its correction lies within the area of established balanced body chemistry which is controlled by the endocrine glands.

Dr. Perera found that twice as many women as men suffer from high blood pressure. Also, more women tend to be overweight than men. The average age at which hypertension can be detected is about thirty-two, whereas proven cases of its onset beyond the age of fifty are so rare, that he believes that if you do not have it before the age of fifty, you will never have it. Pregnancy and the menopause have little to do with causing or affecting high blood pressure. In many heart and circulatory disease cases, high blood pressure is often present.

High blood pressure and low blood pressure are considered together, for strange as it may seem, their primary causes are similar in that they are both due to abnormalities of body chemistry. The blood pressure is taken at two levels called the diastolic (between surges of blood from the heart) and the systolic (when the pressure of the surge is the highest). It is the latter that is usually considered to be the blood pressure. The normal figure is thought to be from about 105 to 120 and should not increase with age. There is more variation in the pressure from day to day and from one part of the day to another than is commonly known. Pressure may fall as low as 100 in the morning and be 20 or more points higher in the afternoon of the same day.

Increased blood pressure is generally due to one or both of two conditions. The conditions are: 1, increased resistance to the blood flow through the capillaries due to deposits in the walls of the arteries or 2, increased tension of the arterioles due to maladjustment of the nervous system.

Both of these conditions are due to faulty body chemistry. High diastolic blood pressure generally occurs with a high phosphorus level of the blood and low pressure with a high calcium level of the blood which later increases the systolic pressure.

Low blood pressure is generally caused by insufficient tension of the walls of the arterioles and venous capillaries due to maladjustment of the autonomic or automatic nervous system. Proper nutrition often does much to correct both high and low blood pressure. Sugar and white flour should be omitted from the diet and the trace minerals added. When high pressure is due to nervous tension it tends to lower quite rapidly under this treatment. To remove the calcium deposits usually takes longer, the phosphorus level must be raised to the point where there is no longer free or excess calcium in the blood. This means that the glandular function must be restored to normal. This may take several months or several years, depending upon the ability of the body to respond to the more efficient chemical conditions.

Posterior pituitary hormone deficiencies are responsible in my opinion for some of the hypertension, some of the cataracts, much of the dental decay, and a good deal of the tendency toward spontaneous abortion. Habitual drinking, pyorrhea and other forms of arthritis also can be traced to this deficiency.

Extreme cases of impaired function of the posterior pituitary gland results in diabetes insipidis, and the sugar metabolism becomes impaired also. There are many causes of impaired function of the posterior pituitary gland which go unrecognized. Much of the so-called essential hypertension is the result of imbalance of the posterior pituitary gland and the adrenal cortex.

People suffering from an overactive anterior pituitary gland may also be quite subject to heart trouble. Usually these people give a history of duodenal ulcer, cancer, heart trouble or diabetes in their family tree. Unless corrected, this hyper anterior pituitary gland can be expected to produce the same pathology in the person as existed in his forbear with the same endocrine situation. Many of these people die of coronary occlusion at the climacteric, right at the time of their greatest value to mankind. This will continue until it is recognized by the profession that such an outcome is avoidable. Such occurrences are possibly the greatest of tragedies resulting from a lack of knowledge of a person's predisposition to pathology.

Another important factor in causing hardening of the arteries or ulceration of the arteries is a too high cholesterol level in the blood. Many people do not understand that cholesterol is a normal part of any human body and must be present, in the right amount, to insure good health. Cholesterol forms the raw material from which the body manufactures vitamin D, bile salts and the adrenal hormones. Although little understood, cholesterol must be of vital importance as it is found concentrated in such vital tissues as the brain and nerves. It is produced by all the cells of the body.

After reading the newspapers and particularly the obituary columns, a person can hardly escape the conclusion that he, along with the majority of the population, may be destined to pass away with a heart attack. He is told about the danger of this occurring if his blood pressure is too high, and to prevent this he must be sure that the cholesterol in his blood is not allowed to become so concentrated that masses or deposits of it will clog his blood vessels. He is warned by many well meaning people that he should avoid certain foods, but it seems that each person has a different idea about the foods to be shunned. Finally he reaches a state of confusion and hardly knows what he should or should not eat—in fact he begins to wonder if he might be better off not eating at all. Truly some of the diets which are recommended amount to just about that as far as the nourishment and food value they supply are concerned.

Since it has been reliably estimated that perhaps fifty per cent or more of the population of the United States, Canada, and Western Europe may be affected by atherosclerosis before reaching the age of fifty, the concern over cholesterol levels can be well understood.

Because of a great desire to do something that might help the person with a dangerously high cholesterol level, both drugs and special diets have been tried. Often the results have been unsatisfactory.

It is believed by many that the condition of atherosclerosis arises because of ill chosen or excessive intake of lipids, and that its development and consequences can be delayed or escaped by selection or adjustment of the intake of cholesterol or fat. This idea derives some support from laboratory findings that animals not afflicted with the disease, after eating large amounts of cholesterol, produce deposits not unlike those found in human atherosclerosis. In spite of this, detailed study of advanced cases of humans has provided no incriminating evidence as to the part diet has played in the condition. Trials of various modifications of fat intake for the present are to be regarded as entirely empiric.

Two types of diet are now in frequent use. One attempts avoidance of cholesterol, with or without strict limitations of fat intake. The other emphasizes limiting fat intake with avoidance of overweight, but without great emphasis upon the amount of cholesterol in the diet.

To most patients, these diets represent a hardship which seems useless since there is little benefit to be derived. Careful observations have been made on the effect of varying the amount of cholesterol in the diet. It was found that even complete avoidance of cholesterol foods did not really change the concentration of the cholesterol in the serum. Likewise single ingestion of large amounts of cholesterol had very little influence upon the cholesterol levels.

As early as 1953 it was reported in *The American Journal of Medicine* that diet, and the eating of foods high in cholesterol, especially fats, seemed to be of very little importance, if any, in influencing cholesterol levels. Although mechanical factors may play a role in the cause of atherosclerosis, these factors are usually influential in determining the sites where the deposits will be made, and in accelerating the rate of lipid disposition at these sites, rather than in determining the cholesterol levels in blood.

It is widely accepted now that the basic cause is in the nature of metabolic defect. It is now known that the body itself makes cholesterol from compounds derived from fats, proteins, and carbohydrates. It is surely understandable from this how impossible it is to control the body cholesterol by avoiding either fat or cholesterol in foods.

In fact, many people have no doubt injured their health by avoiding fat because fat is necessary for the maintenance of a healthy body. However, hydrogenated fats, which are semi-artificial fats in that after being hydrogenated, are in a form that does not exist in a natural state and cannot be easily handled by the body. Other factors of diet seem to play a part on cholesterol levels, but these fall within the realm of the unnatural foods, stimulants, or "empty calories." The results of research, carried on by Dr. Callie Mae Coons and Dr. Madelyn Womack in feeding rats on a sugar plus fat combination diet, showed that ordinary table sugar probably plays on important part in the formation of cholesterol, particularly cholesterol in excess. As necessary as cholesterol is, it can be a deadly substance when it accumulates in excessive quantities in places where it does not belong. In other words, those foods which have adverse effect upon the glands indirectly affect cholesterol metabolism. Probably the danger in diet is due to the refined carbohydrates—sugar, candy and all foods made with sugar—and the effects of caffeine from drinking coffee, and the "empty calorie" foods all of which upset the normal function of the glandular system. It is also possible that the chemical preservatives and insecticide residues found on most commercially processed foods may play some part. Anything that is a foreign substance to the body, which the body cannot handle in a normal way, usually upsets the proper functioning of the glandular system and this in turn accounts for unbalanced body chemistry of which too high a cholesterol level is one dangerous symptom.

We believe on the basis of experience that a high cholesterol level, like many other imbalances of the human mechanism, can be corrected and controlled by achieving a balance of the body chemistry. We find that cholesterol levels, the same as others such as sodium, calcium, phosphorus, etc., fall into line when the body's chemistry is in correct balance. The body must receive proper nourishment, and this means not only the foods it should have, but also omitting those foods which are harmful. Often it is necessary to correct glandular imbalances that were inherited or acquired through years of wrong living before even a proper diet can be of any assistance. It is amazing, but nevertheless understandable, how quickly the cholesterol level returns to normal after the correct amounts of the necessary hormones for each individual are given. It is impossible for the body to function properly with the glandular system out of balance. Remember that the endocrines control ALL of the body's chemistry. Doctors who know little or nothing about the role endocrines play in changing cholesterol levels, have been amazed at the results achieved simply by establishing a correct body chemistry. Often they had labored unsuccessfully to bring about this change through the use of different diets or medications to little or no avail. They are especially dumbfounded to learn that the patient had avoided neither fat nor cholesterol foods. It does seem like magic, but the body can perform amazing feats if it is put in the right working order.

Two typical cases of patients successfully treated through the body chemistry approach are given as follows: a hard driving business man of fifty-five had for several years been suffering from hardening of the arteries and heart disease in general. His diet was that of the ordinary American type with great amounts of coffee, sugar and foods containing sugar, white flour and milk. His body measurements showed that he had a slightly underactive posterior pituitary gland, a highly overactive anterior pituitary function and an overactive production of male hormones. He was too andric and presented the type of graph common to heart attack victims. His blood pressure was slightly high. He was put on the Page Diet and given a minute dosage of estrogen, insulin and adrenal cortex as determined by complete blood analyses. His improvement was rapid, and as long as he follows the prescribed program and especially the natural, wholesome diet, he will probably suffer no further difficulties.

The second case is that of the president of a large electronics distributing corporation, who at fifty-seven had already suffered a brain hemorrhage, circulatory difficulties and had a bad vascular condition in general. His endocrinograph showed that he was the type of individual who is predisposed to heart and circulatory trouble. He had overactivity of the thyroid, anterior pituitary and male hormone producing glands. In his case, all he needed to establish sound body chemistry was minute dosages of estrogen suitable to the requirements of his body and to follow the Page Diet. He is now getting along fine and states that he never felt better or enjoyed his work more. In each of these cases discussed, cholesterol and blood pressure levels returned to normal with the establishment of balanced body chemistry. All patients are given natural mineral and vitamin supplements just to make sure that they are receiving these vital necessities for sound health.

It has been well established that smoking is not a healthful habit, but for heart attack victims, it is even more dangerous, so reported researchers from Wayne State University Medical School early in 1960. In their research, patients volunteered to permit the doctors to work two thin plastic tubes into their hearts and put a hollow needle into the artery of the arm Following three cigarettes, blood pressure and oxygen readings definitely showed that it was necessary for the heart to work much, much harder, although it received little or no extra oxygen. It would be wise for heart attack victims and those people prone to heart attacks, to stop smoking completely. Smoking puts too much stress and strain upon the heart.

Along with coronary troubles, ulcers are one of the

most common of the degenerative diseases. The most common area for ulcers is the duodenum, which is at the outlet of the stomach. It is thought by the profession that worry is a contributing cause, but everyone who worries does not get ulcers.

It is known that an excessive amount of hydrochloric acid is produced by the chief cells of the stomach in such cases, sometimes as much as ten times the normal amount. It is presumed that this abnormal amount of acid irritates and actually digests the stomach lining at the point that hemorrhage takes place, and at times breaks through the stomach walls. This is called a perforating ulcer.

However, the real cause of ulcers is unknown. The remedies at present used are chiefly anti-acids to neutralize some of the acid, the use of milk at two-hour intervals to give the acid something to work on besides the stomach itself, and to dilute the secretions.

The physiology involved is interesting. In a normal person a substance called secretin is formed in the small intestine which goes into the blood and serves to fortify the cells of the stomach against being digested by its own acid. In the case of ulcers, this substance is thought to be insufficient to do so.

We have been fortunate in learning something of great importance about the cause of ulcers, their prevention and cure. The answer is the same as for all degenerative diseases, only this one responds more readily than most to proper treatment.

Our method of determining the endocrine pattern of the patient or the blueprint of the patient's chemical makeup, gave us the clue.

We have found that when this endocrine pattern shows the patient to be more andric than normal, he is subject to certain types of disease. All people have both andric and gynic factors, but not all are evenly balanced in these two factors. It is in those people having an excess of testosterone that these ulcers appear.

The diet, until the ulcer heals, should be bland and may include boiled milk. Otherwise the patient must adhere strictly to the Page Diet according to his special needs. Sugar and coffee and other stimulants are especially bad for ulcer sufferers. In fact, findings made by medical researchers of York City and County Hospitals show that refined sugar in the diet, and not stress and strain as is so often thought, is the major cause for peptic ulcers. The glands are primarily responsible, but in that sugar can throw the glands into complete malfunction, sugar then may probably well be one of the major causes of ulcers. As in all degenerative diseases, diet is important in that it has an effect upon the endocrine glands. Fortunately, healing of ulcers under the Page treatment usually takes only a short time, sometimes just a matter of a very few weeks. Following healing, the patient then adheres to the Page diet and continues to take endocrine supplements if clinical tests indicate their need.

These patients are all hustlers. They have usually made good in the business or professional world. Their andric qualities sustains them until the age of the climacteric. Then they are stricken. Many die between the ages of forty-nine and fifty-four, some even earlier. If they survive the first blow whether it be angina pectoris, heart block, occlusion or thrombosis, their chances of living are still good if the cause is corrected.

But so many are struck without warning. Some even have been pronounced in good physical condition just prior to their heart attack. When the endocrine patterns of people are known to their doctors, many lives will be saved. People do not have to have even the first attack.

This brings up the subject of the male climacteric. If they live long enough, all males go through the climacteric.

In a healthy male with a correct endocrine pattern this change is so gradual that it is just normal aging, but in others with overactive anterior pituitary glands especially, the change is far from placid. It is more like the tempests that rage during the hurricane season. The person going through the climacteric realizes something is wrong with him both physically and mentally. He is emotionally unstable. In his lucid moments he wonders if he is quite right. He is seized with fits of elation and depression. His wife may divorce him. Lucky is the man who has a wife who will stand by him while he is beset by the devil. If she happens to be going through the climacteric at the same time, there is no peace and quiet. This is an excellent reason for a difference in ages of married couples.

And the worst of it is that it often lasts so long. It may be two years, it may be ten. It takes place usually between the ages of forty and sixty. But by maintaining balanced body chemistry during this period, the adjustment can be made rapidly without the perils of perhaps developing ulcers and other degenerative ailments.

It is unfortunate that these discoveries are not generally known among the healing professions. There has been no effort to conceal the methods employed. On the contrary, we have invited and constantly urge any doctor to attend our course in body chemistry and observe the procedure followed, and to use the approach himself in his own practice.

A student of twenty-two years of age, from the local junior college where I usually give several lectures on health yearly, heard one of my lectures and came by the clinic. He had suffered repeatedly from sore and bleeding gums. Treated locally, the condition would clear up only to return within a few weeks. He was plagued with ulcers and had high blood pressure. He is a fine looking, husky young man full of energy and exceptionally well built. A superficial glance would lead you to think him in perfect health. Yet he was already beginning to be plagued with the symptoms of several degenerative diseases. His diet was regularly—sugar, sugar products, white flour, milk, soft drinks, coffee—just the usual American diet that is the best in the world when measured in dollars and cents, but one of the poorest when measured in nutritive value. His endocrinograph showed that both the thyroid and anterior pituitary glands were overactive while the posterior pituitary gland was underactive; this was verified through the blood and urine analyses. He was given three tablets of

1/1200 milligrams of estrogen and three units of insulin daily and put on the Page Diet. Within six weeks all symptoms of his difficulties had disappeared, and he has had no recurrence to date. He reports that he has never enjoyed such fine health. This young man is lucky because he started doing something about his troubles at a young age. He can now expect to live his full life expectancy in good health, because he has learned how to take proper care of his body and the importance of doing so.

Cancer is one of the most prevalent of degenerative diseases. The term cancer covers a wide range of territory, as there are many types of cancer, but all are characterized by cells that have gone crazy in growth and devour healthy cells eventually causing death to the organism. Recent research on the cause of leukemia, often termed blood cancer, sponsored by the American Cancer Society and carried out by Dr. Steven O. Schwarts, representing the Hektoen Institute of Medical Research of Chicago, shows the cause to be a virus. But, Dr. Schwarts emphasized that the virus was like a seed and could not grow unless all conditions were very favorable—good soil and enough sunshine, rain, and warmth. Applied to human beings, this means that a state of body chemistry must be present which favors the virus and makes it possible for it to take hold and grow. This state of body chemistry is controlled by two factors, one heredity, and second, environment, of which diet is an all important part. People who have balanced body chemistry are not subjected to these diseases although they are exposed to them constantly. This has been the message of the pioneering work of Dr. Page for some forty years.

Cancer is one of the greatest causes of death today among people of all ages. According to the American Cancer Society cancer kills more children between the ages of three and fifteen than any other disease. With the incidence of cancer so high, anyone in dental practice is bound to see many cases whether he recognizes them or not. One who does a complete blood chemistry examination as well as making out the endocrine patterns for each patient is bound to arrive at some conclusions over a period of forty years. We have, but first we wish to point out certain facts regarding cancer.

First, cancer cells differ from those from which they originate only in rate of growth and in the abnormal size of the cell.

We have noticed that those cancer cases we have seen had almost invariably overactive anabolic glands. About 95 per cent of these had overactive anterior pituitary glands and abnormally high sugar levels. It is well known that cancer and diabetes are often allied diseases.

Dr. Meyerhof of the University of Pennsylvania believes that the growth of cancer cells might be checked if biochemists could find a way to curb the tumor's appetite for sugar. He finds that fast growing cells such as cancer need an abnormal amount of sugar for their growth as they split the sugar molecule into lactic acid molecules by a process akin to alcoholic fermentation called glycolysis. It is this lactic acid which is essential for the growth of cancer cells. If this could be limited, then growth could be slowed.

We believe that the sugar level of the blood is even more important than Dr. Meyerhof states. We do not remember seeing a single cancer case that had a correct blood sugar level, yet in most non-cancer cases this is easily obtained by means of a sugar-free diet alone.

Furthermore, there are physicians who have had some considerable success with cancer cases by using small doses of insulin. Dr. Beale has successfully used doses of two or three units of insulin two or three times per week together with a proper diet in cancer cases for at least 15 years, to my knowledge. I have used insulin in small amounts to obtain a correct blood sugar level for many patients. Some of these were reported to have cancer. Some of these, if they did have cancer at one time, certainly show no appearance of it now. Our object was not to control the sugar level so much as it was to inhibit the anterior pituitary gland, but the sugar levels of the blood serve as an index of the amounts of insulin or other glandular substance required.

Diet has become an all important factor in its relationship to cancer; this is especially true of the diet characteristic of modern America. Most commercially processed foods are put up with chemical preservatives or other fabrications of the chemical laboratory which are supposed to give the product better qualities for the consumer; however the only benefit gained is actually for the producer. Many of the chemical preservatives, coal tar dyes, artificial coloring, emulsifiers and food additives are highly suspected of being carcinogens—capable of producing or causing cancer. Also, many of the pesticide residues that remain on fruit and vegetables are suspected of causing cancer, and some have been proven to be carcinogens. One cannot always rely upon the pronouncements of the Food and Drug Administration as to how safe these chemical compounds are as they are handicapped by the laws and conditions under which they work. Many of these compounds once thought to be safe and which were approved by the Food and Drug Administration were later found to be very harmful. For example, coumarine was a popular flavor ingredient of cocoa and chocolate products and imitation vanilla extract for seventy-five years before it was determined to be toxic and very dangerous to the lives of test animals. Its use was then prohibited. Very recently the Food and Drug Administration has withdrawn its approval from a number of food dyes, which, though for many years considered acceptable and harmless, have been found to be unsafe and strongly poisonous to human beings as well as animals. The fact that approval was withdrawn when these items were found to be harmful is little comfort to the consumer who may have been using them for years on the assumption that his health was being looked after and safeguarded by highly trained and experienced government chemical, biological, and toxicological experts. Unfortunately, the use of chemical agents is on the increase along with sugar and sugar products,

milk and milk products, coffee, and hydrogenated fats.
Many of these items, particularly the chemical compounds used as preservatives, have been shown to cause
cancer in rats. Many producers laugh at this and say
that this is a rat, but humans are different. Humans are
certainly different, but our physiology is similar; that is
why rats are used as experimental laboratory animals. If
something has a harmful effect upon rats, humans would
be very well advised to never eat it. Possibly the extremely
alarming increase in cancer in the United States is partially
due to the widespread consumption of so many chemical
preservatives, food additives, artificial and synthetic colorings and flavorings, and pesticide residues along with the
modern foods that we eat each day. Even much of our commercial bread has chemical preservatives added. Whole-
wheat bread, which is more nutritive, usually has more
than white bread because whole wheat spoils more rapidly. Actually, of what value are all of these preservatives to
you—the consumer? It is wise to always read the labels on
all processed foods that you buy, and if chemical preservatives, food additives, emulsifiers, artificial flavorings and
artificial colorings are listed, then it would be best to dis-
pense with using the product. These things have an accu-
mulative effect and it may take from ten to thirty years before the harmful effects become noticeable.

Another substance that has been widely used is the synthetic female hormone stilbesterol to put on additional
weight in beef cattle and chickens and promote growth. It
has been proved that stilbesterol can cause cancer in rats
and have other harmful effects. The Food and Drug Administration has prohibited the use of stilbesterol in chickens, but it can still be used, as of the writing of this book,
for cattle and is used quite a bit for beef cattle. Because
the residue of stilbesterol cannot be found in the beef so
treated, it is assumed by the Food and Drug Administration that it is not present. However, more refined techniques may prove its presence as has been the case with
other chemicals long in use and thought to be non-harm-

ful. When that happens, the Food and Drug Administration will, of course, prohibit its use. In the meantime, the wise consumer will not use beef that has been raised with the help of stilbesterol.

All of these agents are foreign to the body, and any foods or chemicals which are foreign agents to the body may be toxic, and if so will probably have such harmful effect upon the glandular system that chemical imbalance may develop as well as presenting a good host to infection.

The role of smoking in lung cancer has been previously pointed out. All of these so-called modern innovations which we indulge in every day, instead of in a moderate manner, probably play their role in making the human body susceptible to degeneration. They form a complex, so to speak, in that not only one foreign agent is taken into the body each day, but a whole series in the form of refined sugar, bread, cake, soft drinks, ice cream, candy, coffee, hydrogenated fats, cookies, tobacco, chemical preservatives and other chemical concoctions of one type or another. The mounting increase of cancer and degenerative diseases in general is the strongest argument that can be presented in favor of a good, natural, wholesome diet such as the Page Diet, which is not rigid and is flexible enough enough to suit the needs, most adequately, for any person.

We are of the opinion that the anterior pituitary gland can become toxic in the same manner that the thyroid gland becomes toxic. Since the anterior pituitary gland manufactures the growth hormone, any lack of control of the pituitary or an abnormal secretion put out by the pituitary gland might produce chaos in the metabolic activities of the cells it was made to regulate.

Another factor which has been almost totally overlooked is the role that milk may play in cancer. To say anything against milk as a food partakes of the nature of heresy. It is accepted by practically everyone, including our best nutritionists, as our most excellent food. Perhaps it is the universal acceptance which protects it from inquiry and investigation. Milk contains the growth hormones which are found in the blood of the animal that manufactures it. This is obvious since milk is made from blood.

The normal animal does not give three or four gallons of milk daily, but very much less than that. Today cows are produced to give greater quantities of milk by endocrine freaks through breeding with that result in mind.

To get this result an overactive anterior pituitary gland is required since that gland produces the lactogenic hormone responsible for milk production. However, it also produces the growth hormone. Now if a person already has a too active anterior pituitary gland, and a history of cancer in his ancestry, he may augment this tendency by drinking milk.

It is said that Switzerland has one of the highest rates of cancer per capita, along with Denmark and the United States. These three places also take the lead in milk production and in the order named.

The Page Foundation Incorporated, dedicated to research in the causes and prevention of degenerative diseases, has a vital interest in the problem. The medical profession, as a whole, is seeking for the answers among the miracle drugs and serums, plus constant dependence upon surgery, x-ray and radium. They have not proven the cause; treatment is too often merely amelioration, and public fear mounts.

Among the findings of the medical profession is the establishment of a relationship between the need for the female hormone, estrogen, to assist in controlling cancer of the prostate in men, and either estrogen or testosterone (the male hormone) to assist in controlling cancer of the breast in women. Published case histories of patients so treated is evidence that the medical profession acknowledges that at least part of the answer to the cause, cure, and prevention of cancer may lie in the field of endocrine dysfunction.

It is our belief that the records accumulating in our files and those of our associates will greatly enlarge the link between cancer and endocrine dysfunction. We do not claim a cure or treatment for cancer; we cannot diagnose its presence through our blood tests; but those who are now reviewing our cases can show definite correlation between endocrine patterns and the presence of a family history of cancer. Furthermore, where correction of inefficiency of body chemistry has been achieved in patients with active cancer, the indirect effects upon the disease are startling and gratifying.

As you well know, cancer strikes in many parts of the body. Among our patients we have cases previously diagnosed by the medical profession as having had cancer of the liver, the blood, the mouth, the skin, cancer of the prostate, the stomach and the intestines. Since our work is not treatment of disease symptoms, but rather correction of the inefficiency of body chemistry, treatment procedure is based on body measurement tests and blood analyses. It consists of corrected diet and inhibition of supplementation of endocrine function as suggested by the endocrine pattern as proven beneficial through correct blood balances.

When maximum efficiency of body chemistry is achieved and maintained, the body's own ability to resist a hostile environment or to cope with previously acquired ills, is amazingly strengthened. What better way is there to illustrate this fact than to report that the cancer of the liver case who was doomed by the medical profession to die within three months is now some years later still living and working happily. The cancer of the mouth patient is reported in good health. The leukemia and the melanoma patient, who five years ago was given only two months to live was instead ordered by her physician to return to work (within a year and a half) and is still going strong. The patient with cancer of the prostate seven years later was found by biopsy to have no further malignancy. The skin cancer has disappeared. The patient with cancer of the intestine, once so serious as to be considered inoperable has survived two operations for obstruction within the past year and is up and about. The cancer of the stomach patient, though a recent one, shows evidence of increased fighting ability within his own mechanism.

Remember, we are not claiming either diagnosis, cure, or treatment of cancer, but we are suggesting, quite pointedly so, that the search for a serum or miracle drug for cancer is not the only source to seek for its cure and prevention; that the use of surgery, x-ray and radium, all destructive of bodily efficiency, may not be the only aid available; that amelioration of cancer symptoms need no longer appease the public; that the answer to the control and prevention of this dreaded scourge may be within the body itself, an improper supply of raw materials (food) and/or a faulty mechanism of utilization (the endocrines).

In our files, in the correlation of our findings, lie invaluable clues for those scientists who are ever alert to see new relationships between already known facts. It is this for which the Page Foundation stands.

Allergies which so often result in asthma, sinusitis, or digestive disturbances, is a common degenerative disease. The symptoms are those typical of glandular dysfunction and nutritional deficiencies, and the cause generally given is "sensitivity to foods, pollens, or dust." Actually the sensitivity is merely a symptom; the real cause lies in the breakdown of the cells in different part of the body. Sometimes this occurs in the mucous membranes of the nose and throat, but more often in the intestinal wall.

Normally the intestinal wall can be permeated by only four substances, sugar, water, the amino and fatty acids, and the mineral salts in solution. Where allergies occur the efficiency of the intestinal wall has been reduced to the point where proteins are able to permeate it and directly enter the blood stream. Treatment, therefore, should not be based on the removal of harmful foods, pollens, and dust except as a temporary measure for the relief of symptoms, but upon the causes of the imperfect body chemistry. In cases of allergies or asthma in children, the addition of the trace minerals often clears up the difficulty with rapidity. In adults, response is slow to diet alone, because the deficiency has been of such long standing that it takes a greater length of time to reestablish normal body chemistry.

The problem of sterility in both women and men is mounting. Already it is estimated that approximately 18 per cent of the women in the United States of child-bearing age cannot have children, and no doubt a good percentage of men are sterile. This of course becomes only a problem to couples when they wish to have a family. Dr. Edith L. Potter, pathologist at the Chicago Lying-In Hospital and professor of pathology in the gynecologic department at the University of Chicago, reports that diet and good nutrition is all important in treating sterility. Some obstetricians have reported excellent results with the use of hormones. During the past twenty-five years, quite a few young married women have come to our clinic seeking establishment of sound body chemistry because they were unable to become pregnant. Sterility and miscarriage are generally caused by dysfunction of the body's glandular system. Many gynecologists are beginning to realize this. In the cases treated for bringing about balanced body chemistry where sterility was one of the problems, the results have been excellent. Also, research carried on by the noted psychiatrist, Dr. E. Gustave Newman of Duke University shows that healthy couples continue to enjoy sexual relations right up into very old age and even into the 90's. He finds that the major reason for the discontinuance of marital relations is ill health. This is of course logical. When the body is healthy, life can be carried on as intended and in an enjoyable manner. The best way, and actually the only way to enjoy sound health is to have balanced body chemistry. Ill health dulls the edge of enjoyable living—it cuts short complete living.

According to an address made by Dr. E. Vincent Askey, who was inaugurated as president of the American Medical Association in 1960, overweight is the nation's greatest health problem. This is probably true because obesity is certainly one of the most obvious signs that the body is not functioning properly—that a state of glandular dysfunction exists. As previously pointed out, this glandular imbalance may be due to bodily constitution having its base in heredity or to a poor diet or both. Usually both factors are involved, but the underlying cause is to be found in inefficient function of the metabolic processes of the body. Most of the thousands of patients who have passed through the Page Clinic lost excess weight when sound body chemistry had been established. More and more the medical profession is coming to realize that overweight is due to faulty body chemistry. Dr. Herbert Pollack, chairman of the American Heart Association's Nutrition Committee, stated in 1959 that there are many factors to be considered in obesity other than just overeating. The problem is one of metabolism, in other words body chemistry. Dr. Pollack stated that research had shown that after the age of twenty-five, the body requires about one per cent less food per year up to a point. One reason for this may be that people also cut their exercise drastically after the age of twenty-five and thus burn up less energy. It is a fact that most people do not exercise enough today. Exercise is well recognized as one aspect of maintaining good health. Dr. Jean Mayer of the Nutrition Department of the Harvard School of Public Health has pointed out that obese people very often inherit a tendency to be overweight. All of these things are coming to be recognized, but the solution to the problem is not generally known. The answer to overweight, which presently afflicts some fifty million Americans and at least eleven per cent dangerously so, is to be found in establishing balanced body chemistry which is done through endocrine supplementation as needed by each overweight person according to his specific needs and following the Page Diet. Most people are prone to think that eating fat makes fat, however, fat does not make fat in the body. A healthy body must have fat to carry on its vital processes. Carbohydrates—the grains, bread, starches, and sugar—are the foods that make fat—and it is these foods that must be curtailed for the person who has great difficulty with obesity. People who wish to lose weight should give up grains, sugar and starches until their desired weight is attained, then they should eat grains and starches only moderately. However, unless balanced body chemistry is brought about, dieting is going to be of very little avail in many cases. There is no specific diet that is good for everyone, or that will work specifically the same for each individual; but as pointed out previously, there are certain foods which are universally harmful to the body and these should never be eaten.

Anyone suffering from overweight is in an unhealthy state which can become acute in time. For each pound of overweight that a person has, five miles of capillaries are required to supply blood to the fat cells. You can imagine the extra stress and strain which is then put upon the heart and circulatory system by each pound of excess weight that the body must support. Also, excess fat cells are not the same as the normal fat cells of the body, all of which points to the fact that overweight is due to a chemical dysfunction of the body. The individual who is obese would be wise to take a sound approach to his problem and act constructively. In our opinion, the only constructive action to take is that of establishing sound, normal body chemistry which will bring about good health and provide insurance against bodily breakdowns that are so characteristic of the prevalent degenerative diseases which are rapidly increasing.

VII.   Dental Decay

Dental decay is the most widespread of the degenerative diseases because it takes only about 25 per cent inefficiency of body chemistry for it to be present. Other degenerative diseases take more inefficiency, but the presence of dental decay clearly shows that further inefficiency will take place in time. Dental decay begins very early in most of our children. The yearly, or twice yearly visit to the dentist has become routine, and many children find it necessary to go much more often. If a child is beset with this degenerative disease at an early age, it is easy to surmise that he will most likely suffer from one of the crippling and killing degenerative diseases sometime during middle age or perhaps even much younger. It is alarming to note the apathy with which the general public regards dental decay; all agree that something should be done about it, but few are willing to look closely at the main causes which are apparent for all to see if they will but look. There has been lots of talk about fluorine in the drinking water lessening dental decay by 10 to 20 per cent, but there are no reliable facts or statistics to back such a claim. Fluorine will not adequately prevent dental decay and it possibly can do real damage to the body. The point is that people don't think in terms of preventing dental decay completely, yet it can be done. The only conclusion that can be drawn is that many people are not interested in preventing dental decay by changing their food habits. The answer lies in diet and body chemistry with diet being the most important factor.

Anthropologists in their study of past civilizations,

primitive peoples, man today and his future, have pointed out that dental decay is a very serious matter indeed and that it is merely a symptom of more serious degeneration in the future. The late internationally famous anthropologist, Dr. E. A. Hooton of Harvard University stated the following:

"I firmly believe that the health of humanity is at stake, and that, unless steps are taken to discover preventives of tooth infection and correctives of dental deformation, the course of human evolution will lead downward to extinction . . . The facts that we must face are, in brief, that human teeth and the human mouth have become, possibly under the influence of civilization, the foci of infections that undermine the entire bodily health of the species and that degenerative tendencies in evolution have manifested themselves in modern man to such an extent that our jaws are too small for the teeth which they are supposed to accommodate, and that, as a consequence, these teeth erupt so irregularly that their fundamental efficiency is often entirely or nearly destroyed.

"In my opinion there is one and only one course of action which will check the increase of dental disease and degeneration which may ultimately cause the extinction of the human species. This is to elevate the dental profession to a plane on which it can command the services of our best research minds to study the causes and seek for the cures of these dental evils . . . The dental practitioner should equip himself to become the agent of an intelligent control of human evolution, insofar as it is affected by diet. Let us go to the ignorant savage, consider his way of eating, and be wise. Let us cease pretending that tooth-brushes and tooth-paste are any more important than shoe-brushes and shoe-polish. It is store food which has given us store teeth."

Dr. Vilhjalmur Stefansson, a noted anthropologist and

world authority on the Eskimo, reports that the Eskimo is 100 per cent free from dental decay as long as he stays on his native diet. Dr. Alex Hrdlicka, for many years the distinguished Curator of Anthropology in the National Museum, Washington, also found that the Eskimo never had dental decay as long as he was on the native diet. But, as soon as he began to eat the American diet which is especially abundant in refined sugar, milk, coffee, white flour and products containing sugar, the Eskimo then began to suffer from rampant dental decay—almost 100 per cent of them then have dental decay. The diet of the Eskimo, which consists almost exclusively of meat (including the fat), not only keeps him free from dental decay, but also gives him perfect jaws and perfectly set teeth. It is easy to see that the Eskimo is free from dental decay because his diet does not create a condition in his body chemistry conducive to degenerative disease.

Many people will say, "Well that is the Eskimo, we are different." Here the anthropologist has data which will prove the contrary. Iceland was settled first by the Irish sometime before 800 A.D. After 850 A.D. the Norsemen came and found the Irish already there. The island had never been settled by any other people. Today the modern Icelander is a mixture of Irish and Norwegian or Scandinavian. These people were isolated from Europe and lived mainly on fish and animal products, ate very little grain, and during the late middle ages had no grain at all. Examination of the skulls of these people have shown that none had dental decay and the examination has been carried out thoroughly by not only anthropologists, but by dentists, physicians, and other scientists as well. Here we have a clear case of a people, who are of the same race as ourselves, completely free from dental decay as long as they remained on a diet rich in fish, meat, and animal products. Today, now that the Icelanders have taken on a diet similar to ours, rich in refined flour and grains, sugar, and coffee, they suffer from about the same percentage of dental decay as we do.

Dr. Weston A. Price, an outstanding pioneer dentist

and a member of the American Physical Anthropology Society, made great contributions to the understanding of dental decay. For many years he had suspected diet as its major cause. He knew of various reports of anthropologists with regard to the lack or near lack of dental decay among many primitive peoples. Dr. Price set off to underdeveloped regions of the world to examine the mouths and teeth of primitive peoples in the Polynesian and Melanesian regions of the South Pacific, Africa, the Americas, and many other regions. His book and great contribution to posterity, *Nutrition and Physical Degeneration,* has become a classic for both dentistry and nutrition. Yet, his findings have been little heeded. In every group that he studied, he found that when the primitive peoples were on their native diet, they were anywhere from 90 to 100 per cent free from dental decay and had perfectly formed mouths. Among the groups who had gone on the civilized diet of Europe and America (namely white flour, coffee, sugar, and sugar-containing products) dental decay became widespread. He has well documented his findings with both statistics and photographs, and anyone would be well rewarded to read his book. Dr. Price knew that diet was responsible for dental decay; he did not discover exactly why that was so. However, he did put me on the right track and it is through the stimulus of Dr. Price that I finally, through many years of patient observation and experimentation, found what that relationship is. Still, diet is basic and most people can be free from dental decay merely by going on a wholesome natural diet.

The co-author of this book, an anthropologist, has done research among the Maya in Yucatan. Earlier studies were conducted by the anthropologist Morris Steggerda and a team of dentists and physicians. Over several years they examined the Maya, making a new examination of the same individual each year. With reference to dental decay, their findings were that the Maya were almost entirely free from dental decay. This survey was taken during the 1930's at a time when the Indians had been little exposed to the European-American diet. Now, the Maya do not have what we would consider the best diet for good nutrition, being short in animal protein; yet they do eat meat whenever they can get it. Their diet is primarily corn and beans with some vegetables and fruit. Yet, on this diet they are almost completely free from dental decay. At that time Dr. Steggerda and his colleagues stated that their immunity to dental decay must be due to their race. However, further studies since then have completely dispelled such an explanation. The Maya who have gone to the city to live and who have taken on the regular civilized diet suffer from rampant dental decay. It should be noted that neither the Maya nor the Eskimo ever brush their teeth. Brushing of the teeth is probably good for general hygience of the mouth and halitosis, but even it can be over done. A hard brush constantly run over the enamel of teeth can actually be harmful. Toothpaste may make the mouth feel good, but its effect in preventing dental decay is very little. The Maya do rinse out the mouth with water after eating. Doesn't it seem a little strange that we, the very civilized, have fancy brushes for cleaning our teeth, which we use constantly with good tasting toothpaste, and yet, we suffer from 98 per cent or more dental decay while the Maya, Eskimo and other primitive groups, who never use these fancy gadgets, are around 90 per cent or more completely free from dental decay. Clearly the answer to preventing dental decay is not to be found in toothpaste and tooth brushes.

The answer to the cause and prevention of dental decay is to be found in nutrition and endocrinology. Some may take exception to the wedding of endocrinology and nutrition in the treatment of dental decay, but the following quotation from the 1935 Report of the Curriculum Survey Committee of the American Association of Dental Schools definitely places systemic correction within the province of our specialty. The report on dental education in the United States and Canada in 1926 pointed out that dentistry should render a comprehensive service in order to meet the health needs of the people, and it suggested that dentistry, expanded as it should be in biological scope and strengthened in its health service aspects, would be devoted:

> To the establishment of the principles and to the application in all forms and degrees, of scientific health service relating directly to the teeth and to the closely adjacent oral tissues, and indirectly to the welfare of other parts of the body and of the whole system (and)
>
> to the discovery of the correlations between dental and oral conditions and systemic diseases, with special reference to observed effects of distant disorders on the teeth and closely adjacent oral tissues, and of dental and oral abnormalties on the health of the body as a whole.

It further states that:

> A diagnosis of oral conditions is not complete without a study of possible signs of impairment of general health and differentiation in signs of local disease from those of systemic disease. The literature of dentistry and medicine contains numerous examples of cases in which diseases of the mouth were treated sometimes for a long time and at great expense, only to find in the end that the problem involved the entire body, not just the mouth alone.
>
> Frequently questions arise between dentists and physicians regarding the diagnosis of oral, particularly dental diseases, physicians sometimes giving a diagnosis and ordering specified dental services. There is a tendency on the part of physicians to refrain from such practices, as dentists become more competent in diagnosis. The public has the right to expect that the dentist will be capable of diagnosing all dental diseases and disorders, for, if he cannot do it, there is no other person to whom the patient can turn.
>
> Closely related to diagnosis in dental service is adequate treatment planning. Treatment, like diagnosis, should take the entire oral situation into consideration, as well as systemic conditions when they may be involved.
>
> The dentist may be regarded as rendering adequate

dental service to his patients if he is competent in these matters. Since the publication of this report there has been a growing tendency to disregard the limitations of one's specialty and to visualize the clinical conditions as an end result dependent upon changes in normal physiology and body chemistry of the organs of a living body which is essentially one unified whole.

It is for these reasons that in my discussion of the problem of dental decay I must of necessity consider other ills as part of the whole picture. In my work I have found a definite interrelated casual relationship between dental decay and other systemic conditions. The mouth is an indicator of health because the presence of degenerative disease can first be detected there. In fact all so-called degenerative diseases—diabetes, arthritis, and those diseases dependent upon the breakdown of some part within the organism—respond to the same type of systemic treatment as dental decay. All seem to be founded upon a reduced chemical efficiency of the body due principally to a lack of adequate building materials.

For some time it has been suspected by the profession that dental decay was indicative of nutritional deficiency. But not until the discovery of the correct interpretation of calcium-phosphorus tests of the blood plasma was this substantiated, and the mechanism understood by which nutritional deficiencies have their effect upon the structure of teeth and the defensive mechanism by which teeth resist decay.

Dentine, the bony structure of the teeth, depends for its well-being upon its nourishment. If it is not well nourished, it is soft; if it is well nourished, it is hard and dense and resistant to bacterial invasion. Not only does the dentine depend upon its nourishment for the internal factors which inhibit disease, but the external environment is affected as well by the state of well-being of the body as a whole. These external environmental factors include the buffer action of the saliva which in turn results from the state of efficiency of the internal factors. Generally, the composition of saliva is not altered by diet, but it does vary in the same direction as changes take place in the blood with respect to blood calcium, phosphate, sodium and potassium levels. The buffer action of saliva is dependent upon the mineral content which is derived from the blood. Thus the blood levels of calcium and phosphorus determine resistance to decay from both the internal and external standpoint.

Correction of dietary factors involved in an adequate nutrition does not necessarily correct the nutrition, for nutrition implies the supplying of the necessary food materials to the tissues within the body. If the assimilation is not efficient, the digestive system may contain the necessary ingredients of good nutrition, yet the blood stream, which supplies these ingredients to the tissues, may be deficient in them.

It is therefore necessary to know how this assimilation may be made to function normally. To do so, a knowledge of the function of glands, exocrines and endocrines, is essential so that any functional inadequacy may be improved by the replacement of glandular substances or by other appropriate means. Actual treatment is temporary, for with proper dietary correction regeneration of endocrine function is to be expected. Just how long it will take for this regeneration varies with the individual. Fortunately there is no guesswork involved, as the calcium-phosphorus tests show exactly how much progress in this direction is being made.

It is apparent that the body uses a compound composed of calcium and phosphorus to supply teeth and bones with nourishment. What ratios of calcium and phosphorus are necessary at the point where they precipitate or act is uncertain, for the parts played by magnesium, sodium, and potassium are unknown as well as the acid-alkaline point of deposit. The answer has been found and proven by a comparison of my analyses with some 40,000 clinical findings. It was found that a constant ratio of calcium and phosphorus (10-4) in the blood plasma is the optimum requirement of adults with a higher and varying level of phosphorus requirement for growing children, and lower but still proportional levels of both being required in old age. And so we come to the conclusion that although the ratios of calcium and phosphorus at the point of bone manufacture remain unknown, the process is dependent upon the presence of a certain proportion of these minerals in the blood.

The bones and teeth are known to serve as a storehouse of calcium and phosphorus to be added to in times of plenty, and to be subtracted from in times of scarcity. On the basis of some 40 thousand blood tests taken during the past 30 years, we can state that in clinical cases in the adult, the critical point is reached when the calcium shows 8.75 mg. per 100 cc of blood and when the phosphorus shows 3.5 mg. per 100 cc of blood. Below these amounts for either calcium or phosphorus, there is a withdrawal of minerals from the dentine and bone, and above these amounts a reserve is maintained.

For a long time dentists had been suspecting that sugar caused dental decay and much of the circumstantial evidence signaled it as the culprit. As an example, the following experience with patients shows the bad effect of sugar upon teeth through affecting the calcium-phosphorus levels of the blood.

A young, married woman came to me shortly after having finished her hospital training. She appeared with two cavities and several cervical areas of incipient caries. I was interested in determining the reason for them. Her diet was investigated and found to be good, although she was concealing one bad item which was discovered later. She had a nearly perfect set of beautiful teeth. Her metabolism test was excellent but her blood phosphorus was not normal. During the course of the following year about twenty cavities were filled and several blood readings were taken at short intervals. A great deal of attention was paid to her diet. Cod-liver oil, trace minerals, citrus fruit, milk and green leafy vegetables were present but still the decay progressed. Suddenly her phosphorus level went abnormally high for no reason that could be understood. This gave her a usable product of calcium and phosphorus of 36, although throughout the previous year her usable product varied between 21 and 25. (A usable product of at least 30 is necessary to maintain immunity to decay.) Then the answer was found. The patient explained that after she became married she acquired the habit of eating candy, an estimated quarter pound daily. Doubtless this was a reaction to her rigorous hospital training. She concealed this fact until she was sure every other measure of stopping her decay was ineffective. In the succeeding year, candy and sugar being omitted, she had no further tooth decay.

Another girl, a nurse in training, whose blood tests I had taken every three months and who had been immune to caries for a year, suddenly developed two cavities together with a drop in her phosphorus to an abnormal level. She had spent the previous six weeks in the diet kitchen and during that time hardly ever ate a regular meal but she satisfied her hunger with cakes and sweets whenever the spirit moved her. At the end of her dietary spree and after her dental work had been completed she ceased developing further cavities.

These two experiences led me to undertake experiments with sugar. Subjects of whom I had numerous blood tests were selected. Immediately after taking a blood sample, each was given all the candy she wanted and other blood tests were taken at intervals. There was no change in two hours, but in two and one-half hours the phosphorus level dropped five-tenths of a milligram This was after eating nine pieces of chocolate candy—one-fourth of a pound. This was enough to make a difference of nine points in the usable product of calcium and phosphorus. It can easily be seen that if this were continued daily, decay would be active in these people.

Besides cavities, we have other oral diseases which are related to systemic conditions. Calculus deposits are found to be coincident with a high calcium level. These deposits were found to be greater in proportion when there was an excess of calcium above the amount which would combine with the phosphorus present. When a ratio of 10 of calcium and 4 of phosphorus was obtained, there was no evidence of calcular deposits. Therefore, the assumption is that calcium greater in amount than can be used by the phosphorus is more or less free calcium, and is excreted through secretions made from the blood, one of which is the saliva. Another fact noted was the presence of serumnal calculus and irritated gums when the phosphorus level was more than 40 per cent of the calcium level. When the phosphorus level was reduced this irritation or gingivitis often cleared up without surgical interference. This does not indicate that surgical interference is unnecessary when there are serumnal or salivary calculus deposits. It means only that both local and systemic treatment should be used together rather than either separately.

The alveodar ridges are those bony structures upon which we rest artificial dentures. They are subject to the same chemical laws and require the same constituents as dentine. The continued satisfaction of dentures is dependent upon the stability of these supports. If, however, these ridges are changing due to chemical imbalance, no dentures will give permanent satisfaction. So those of you who suffer from ill fitting dentures should look to your diet.

Pyorrhea, an inflamed condition of the gums, generally occurs when the glands are malfunctioning, causing a high phosphorus level. By reducing the phosphorus to its proper relation to calcium, inflammation can be eliminated. Pyorrhea and the usual form of dental decay are opposed to each other. We do not find both in the same patient at the same time. Pyorrhea is a form of arthritis; a different nomenclature is used merely because of the location of the symptoms. Bone tumors (hyperostosis) are quite common among those with dentures as well as among those who still retain their own teeth.

Erosion is due to two factors—one internal, one external. Decalcification of the surface or enamel of the teeth is due to a mineral imbalance of the saliva. Repeated tests have proven that mineral imbalance of the saliva is merely a reflection of calcium-phosphorous imbalance of the blood; when the calcium-phosphorus levels are brought into a normal ratio in the blood, the salivary secretions are no longer acid and erosion disappears.

Electrolysis occurs when there are fillings of two different metals in the mouth and the body's chemistry is out of balance. When the body's chemistry is normal, however, no electric current is set up between the different metals. To illustrate an instance of electrolysis, pyorrhea and their interrelationship with other bodily ills of a deficiency nature, we will consider a case of tropical sprue which recently came to our attention:

Mr. D. a man of about forty-five, 5'6" in height and weighing 128 pounds told me that he had sprue. A dental examination disclosed pyorrhea, electrolysis, and a history of considerable decay. His blood pressure was 115/70, and his phosphorus level was high in proportion to the calcium. Mr. D. thought rapidly but spoke with hesitation. His color was very bad (a pasty grey) and his eyes were dull and red-rimmed. Acute inflammation of the entire intestinal tract, a sore tongue and mouth plus the electrolysis made him most uncomfortable. He had followed the bland diet usually recommended for sprue and had received temporary relief from his symptoms. Unfortunately, after a few months his difficulties returned worse than before. His endocrinograph indicated glandular imbalance. Daily insulin treatment of three unit doses was prescribed, the trace minerals were added to his diet and sugar was eliminated. He was put on the Page Diet. Within a few weeks Mr. D's eyes brightened, the speech hesitation gradually lessened, the redness about his eyes disappeared and he began to add to his diet those foods which he had been unable to eat for some years: that is, butter, potatoes and bread. The pyorrhea began to clear up and although the electrolysis and sore tongue came and went, the periods of relief from these grew longer. The calcium-phosphorus levels began to approach normal. The disease, of course, was of such long standing, the symptoms so acute and numerous, that it took several months to secure complete cessation of symptoms and longer to attain real health. But please note that the same treatment used for pyorrhea and electrolysis was effective in caring for the symptoms of sprue. All were due to systemic conditions. By correcting body chemistry, relief was obtained from both oral and other bodily symptoms.

Just as inflammation of a tooth joint is known to dentists as pyorrhea, while inflammation of any other joint is known to physicians as arthritis, so do we find parallels in other diseases of the mouth and the rest of the body. The physician treats a certain condition by one method, the dentist treats it by a second method and neither has the advantage of the other's experience.

In yet another way does lack of common understanding in the professions prove deleterious to the patient. Without an understanding of nephritis, the dentist's efforts in treatment of pyorrhea may prove futile. Acute arthritis of the foot may have its bearing on a stubborn case of gingivitis. Inflammation anywhere in the body will influence the outcome of inflammatory or infectious conditions of the mouth.

The condition of oral mucosa often furnishes important diagnostic information. The membrane of the cheek, the lips, the gingiva and especially the tongue often present symptomatic changes, the correct interpretation of which may lead to the discovery of serious bodily diseases. These in turn form a background for lesions in the mouth which usually resist local treatment as long as the metabolic disturbance remains unrecognized and thus untreated.

Even cases of injury to body healing ability may be related to dental conditions. A certain patient had as he expressed it, never a sick day in his life until he was in an automobile accident. He spent the next three years and his life savings trying to get well. Eleven operations failed to close a fistula. Finally a new physician suggested that a dentist look at his mouth. After the removal of seven devitalized teeth, the fistula closed and the man became well.

There are several remedies and methods of treatment used by the dentist for dry socket. If, however, the dentist realized that dry sockets are really a form of osteomyelitis he would have the advantage of the experience of many physicians and surgeons in his efforts to cope with the problem. If both physicians and dentists understood more of the systemic predisposing causes of dry socket and osteomyelitis, both would be more successful in treatment. Both diseases take place at the site of injury, but only when the predisposing causes are present. A predisposing cause is a low level of calcium in the blood and high phosphorus, which in turn is the result of inefficient body chemistry.

Insulin is of great value in treating these conditions. A number of physicians are using three unit daily doses in cases of osteomyelitis with beneficial results. It raises the calcium level and lowers the phosphorus which causes the inflammation to subside. Contrary to popular belief, insulin has many uses other than for diabetes.

The diseases causing the most serious oral disturbances are the vitamin deficiencies, endocrine imbalance, uremia and diabetes. Diabetes can be suspected when teeth decay rapidly or when there is rapid absorption of bony ridges. If the patient also has recent dimming of his vision, and a dry glistening mucous membrane, this diagnosis is even more certain. The presence or absence of sugar in the urine is not to be entirely relied upon. The sugar level of the blood is of great diagnostic value. Most cases of the types encountered by the dentists are sub-clinical in nature and are not easily recognized as diabetes. For this reason it is of great importance to discover them early when prognosis is favorable for a complete recovery through nutritional correction. The patient whose dentist has discovered his incipient diabetes is more fortunate. He will often be frightened enough by the information to follow the rules of nutrition and thus increase his life expectancy over that of the seemingly well, but uninformed person.

Dental caries and osteomalacia result from an insufficient level of combined calcium and phosphorus in the blood. Nutrition is chiefly responsible for adequate or inadequate levels of these minerals. The nutrition may be inadequate because of insufficient essentials in the diet or because of the inclusion in the diet of sugar and coffee.

A long continued inadequacy of the diet may affect the efficiency of the endocrines. In such a case, correction of the diet does not immediately restore the nutrition. The endocrines must respond favorably before the nutrition does, for the endocrines control assimilation.

By successive calcium-phosphorus tests of the blood, the success or failure of dietary correction to influence dental conditions will be noted. In case of failure, supplemental endocrine treatment is indicated. In turn, correctness or incorrectness of the selection of endocrine products, and the amounts of each to be used, are indicated by repetition of these same tests.

The usable calcium-phosphorus levels of the blood make environmental conditions of the teeth favorable or unfavorable for tooth decay. The environmental factors are internal and external. The internal factors control the density and resistance of the dentine to decay, and upon the external factors (buffer action of the saliva) depends the ability to neutralize acids of fermentation. Thus the predisposing causes of dental decay involve the whole body while inciting causes are bacterial. The bacterial causes require local treatment but the systemic causes require treatment based on a study of the functioning ability of the glands of the body.

Thus it was through this approach that I made the discovery of what caused not only tooth decay but the other degenerative diseases as well. After seeing many of my patients, as well as those of my fellow dentists, return year after year with the same old complaint of dental decay, I became determined to find the answer of how to prevent it. The dentist should be a physician whose major interest is in curing and preventing, not just repairing the same old ailments year after year until finally the teeth are gone. Fortunately, dental decay, as well as the other degenerative diseases, can be prevented primarily by two procedures that must go together.

1. Follow a natural diet which eliminates sugar and sugar products, coffee, refined grains (white flour), and milk. (See chapter Four on diet and nutrition.)
2. If there is malfunction of the glands, correction of it.

For most people and children, diet alone is usually sufficient to prevent dental decay. For others, glandular supplement and correction of diet are needed together for various lengths of time.

VIII. Marriage Patterns and Family Life

To judge from the number of unhappy marriages and divorces each year, it is evident that one of the pressing needs of our times is sound and productive marriage counseling. Within this area a great deal has been accomplished from the sociological and psychological points of view. These are very important, but one of the basic aspects in this whole area of human understanding is to be found in the endocrine patterns of the marital partners. Scientists and physicians alike agree that endocrinology holds the key to understanding and prevention of many of the maladies that plague an individual. As important as the endocrine glands are in our emotions, nothing is done in this vital area of marriage counseling, where the malfunctioning of the endocrine glands may account for the troubles. Yet an understanding of such factors can often result in resolving these difficulties.

We are physically, emotionally, and mentally governed by our endocrine glands. Endocrine patterns dictate personalities. Does your chemical makeup produce explosions or peace? This depends in part on your mental control, in part on the mental control of those with whom you associate, but in greater part it depends on the chemical makeup of those whom you contact. Some chemicals can be mixed in a laboratory with excellent results, others with most unhappy or even disastrous aftermaths. So it is with people. Better than explosions or mental control is understanding of the differences in chemical makeup between one person and another, and how these differences may be expressed in the personality.

The physical aspect of a person and his emotional disposition tells us a great deal about his glandular structure.

Let us see—and read what we see—when we look at an obese person. First of all the excessive fat advertises the fact that there is something wrong with the metabolism of this person. Metabolism is controlled entirely by the endocrine glands. He stores up fat because his chemical machinery is inefficient; he does not use his food properly. The controllers of his chemical machinery—of food utilization—are the glands. The placement of the excess fat indicates which glands are functioning abnormally. If he is heavy all over and has a bull neck, he is probably making too much male hormones; he will have a great deal of energy which is characterized by great drive in himself and a tendency to drive others, which is often annoying. If he has a spare tire around the middle, the anterior pituitary is probably underactive. When his weight is primarily in the thighs, with a dip a little below the hip sockets, the posterior pituitary is most likely underactive. When he has an extra large bulge at the calf of the leg and loss of thinning of hair at the center point at the back of the head, there is further indication of posterior pituitary deficiency. When the leg is quite thick just above the ankle an under-active thyroid is indicated.

People with these physical characteristics will tend to have little energy and hence are said to be lazy; they are heavy eaters, and are hard to get along with unless they have the heavy neck indicating too much maleness. Too much maleness will still provide energy and drive, but the underactive anterior pituitary will probably give either a very large appetite or a craving for sweets. A low blood sugar is often found with this type of person. In other words, this type of individual has the energy but becomes exhausted very rapidly, and is tense and irritable.

In contrast with the obese person, let's look at the thin individual. First of all the excess of skin surface in proportion to weight indicates wasted energy thrown off in the form of heat. If the eyes bulge and/or the hair recedes over the eyes, the man probably has an overactive thyroid. A quick temper goes with this type of individual. You will also note in this person a trim, thin ankle. When there is a marked inward dip at the back of and just below the knee, this person may have an overactive anterior pituitary. This will give the individual drive, but he will not always have the physical stamina to back up his ambition and ability, with the result that he may manifest considerable frustration. If this person has underactive adrenal glands, the legs will be thinner at the midcalf than is normal. This type of person cannot stand very much stress, especially between the ages of forty-five and forty-eight.

If you will observe shadings and combinations of the extremes described for the fat person and the thin person, you can learn much concerning their disposition, temperament, and general makeup. You will understand a little more about what makes them "tick," what makes them "different," what makes them "react the way they do," what their "limitations" may be, and their "potentialities." You will understand that what lies at the basis of these things is the function of the endocrine glands. As illustrated above, body form, what the anthropologist calls morphology and somotology—physical types—tells us a great deal about an individual, and defines specific things to the specialist.

Opposites do attract! If this is your first marriage your mate may have an endocrine pattern which is opposite to your own. Nature's prime interest does not seem to be for you, but for your children; therefore, she seems to bring together two persons with contrasting endocrine patterns for the purpose of producing more nearly perfect offspring. There are several combinations of endocrine patterns which will achieve this goal. Consequently, we find that a person with a nearly normal endocrine pattern will tend to marry another with a nearly normal one. However, the andric type person will often marry the gynic type person, and those having an overactive function of certain specific glands will choose a partner having an underactive function of those same glands. While this promises the best possible progeny, it often creates personality conflicts between the marital partners.

Do you have a mate who is quick thinking, quick tempered, and at times tends to be impatient with you? Or does this picture of the overactive thyroid person describe you? If so, we expect your mate to have an underactive thyroid, to be easygoing, even-tempered and a little slower in thought and action than yourself. These characteristics of personality depend to a large degree upon the individual glandular pattern, and a balance of these characteristics between marital partners makes for a happier marriage.

Usually, a person having an overactive function of the posterior pituitary gland will chose a mate having an underactive function of this gland. Not infrequently, however, we do find marriages where both husband and wife have underactivity of the posterior pituitary gland. Apparently this dysfunction shared by both man and wife does not lead to disharmony between them, as it appears to be related to their sexual accord. Nevertheless, such mates unfortunately may produce children who have even greater dysfunction of this important gland. To offset this somewhat, the remainder of the parental graphs may be quite different. For instance, take the case of a young doctor whose endocrine pattern indicates a normal thyroid, underactive posterior pituitary and overactive anterior pituitary, whereas his wife's endocrine pattern shows a normal thyroid, underactive posterior pituitary and underactive anterior pituitary. They are a very happy married couple and have a wonderful family. Their endocrine patterns and their personalities balance each other.

A husband having an overactive anterior pituitary is the type who is a "driver." He drives himself harder than anyone else. He has all the push and ambition needed to be very successful in his chosen business or profession. These men often die at an early age leaving young, attractive, but lonely widows. In fact this drive and ambition becomes in some such an obsession, that although they may achieve high position and amass great sums of money, few of them ever really enjoy life. These men usually have wives who long for a little less ambition, and a little more companionship from their husbands. The wives are less ambitious and desire a slower life, especially if, as endocrine opposites of their husbands, they have underactive pituitary glands.

Now we come to the most complex and least understood of these basic differences, the relationship between the andric type person and the gynic type person. Every individual normally produces both male and female sex hormones. When these are in proper physiological balance, we have a male or female who tends to select a mate having similar good balance. When we find the male or female who produces slightly more of the male type hormone than the average male or female, we consider that person to be "andric." The female or male who produces slightly more female type hormone than the average female or male is termed "gynic." We are not in any sense speaking of the masculine type woman or the feminine type man who are such extremes of andricity and gynicity as to be considered abnormal. The terms "andric" and "gynic" refer to the ordinary people around you living normal lives.

In nearly all first marriages we find the andric type person selecting the gynic type person and vice versa. However ideal this may be for nature's balance, many marital problems are due to this basic difference. The andric male is similar to the overactive anterior pituitary male described above; in fact the andric male very often has overactivity of the anterior pituitary which further accents his andricity. He is usually ambitious, aggressive, a logical thinker, and a leader in his chosen field. He makes the major decisions in the family, often without consulting his wife. She will be a very gynic person, whose major interests lie in the home and her children. She may enjoy social functions, music, fine arts and is apt to be a very creative and sensitive person. Her way of solving problems is based on her own method of intuitive thinking which is no less intelligent, but often highly irritating and nearly always misunderstood by her direct and logical thinking husband.

A relationship producing even greater conflicts is the marriage between the andric woman and gynic man. This marriage has two strikes against it before it starts, and if it does not end in divorce, often results in tragic warping of personalities. Here we have the andric woman who has leadership qualities, ambition, an analytical type of mind, and the gynic man who is nonaggressive and often quite content with the status quo.

Unfortunately, the andric woman tends to dominate her husband and ambitiously drives him. He may permit and even encourage his wife's domination, but he is at a loss to understand his wife's zealous ambition for him since it is not part of his own nature. He feels pushed and inadequate.

The wife, in such a marriage, may be equally unhappy. What she really wants is a husband who takes the lead. Of course traditionally, this is thought to be the ideal relationship between a man and a woman. If the andric wife is not employed, or does not have some activity which provides a constructive outlet for her qualities of leadership, she becomes even more frustrated with her inability to make her husband over into the image of herself. In this type of marriage both the man and the wife are dissatisfied. Another example, though less common, is when two andrics marry. Andrics like to dominate all situations and usually neither mate is willing to give in to the other. This is the andric drive, due to too much male hormone in each mate, that lies at the base of their marital troubles. You have heard this type of couple described as follows: "they get along like cats and dogs—constantly at each other's throat." In cases like this, it is wise for them to decide between themselves that each one will have jurisdiction within certain specified areas, and above all they must understand why they are as they are. Also, by a little glandular supplement, both parties can be usually rendered normal. For example, take the case of two andrics who had been married for a number of years. In their own words, their marriage had been one of continual quarreling because each was determined to have his or her way. The initials of this couple happen to be H and L. Upon understanding their problem, their response, in their own words, was a note signed as follows: "H—L, thanks for taking the EL out of the center." They are now happy as larks and thoroughly enjoying life together. With understanding and treatment, a marriage that seemed to be slated for the divorce courts may now be described as ideal.

Dissatisfaction need not necessarily be the result of this type of marriage provided understanding and intelligence are used by both marital partners. If a man recognizes andric quantities in his wife, he should assist her in finding an outlet for them. If a wife recognizes gynic qualities in her husband and understands her tendency to dominate and take the lead, she will welcome an opportunity to express these qualities in herself elsewhere. Furthermore, if she is intelligent enough to realize that this type of man best fulfills her needs as she fulfills his, then she will guide and cooperate with him in making the major decisions in the family. She will give her gynic husband the appreciation he needs to bring forth his extremely fine qualities, for he is often a sensitive, creative type of individual with much to contribute to the world.

A person with an overactive thyroid gland is quick and alert mentally, but he may be explosive emotionally. You put two overactive thyroids together and there may be fireworks; for example, a mother and son. Until the son is about 12 the relationship with his mother may be satisfactory—he does as he is told. However, at about the age of twelve he begins to assert his masculinity. Possibly she unconsciously objects to this sign of growing maturity the indication that her child will be growing away from her. Friction develops and both tend to lose their tempers simultaneously. If such situations are repeated the mother and the son grow apart. How much better if mother and son discussed the inherent danger of emotional tension between two overactive thyroids, and agreed not to lose their tempers at the same time. With intelligent understanding, the previously good relationship between these two people could be maintained and actually improved; both would grow in maturity.

A different problem may arise between a dominating mother and an andric daughter. The mother might be gynic with an underactive thyroid, anterior and posterior pituitary gland. As a young bride she might have been slim and appealing, but with increasing years would come the middle-age spread and a development of a "Mrs. five-by-five." The low blood sugar which may occur with an underactive anterior pituitary could be one factor tending towards overweight. The mother, dissatisfied with herself, her own lack of drive, her own appearance, might easily take a dominating attitude towards her daughter. The andric daughter, however, as she grew up, would become increasingly antagonistic toward the dominance of a mother who was motivated by emotions rather than logic. The andric child with an overactive posterior pituitary and anterior pituitary would be fully capable of making her own decisions on the basis of logical reasoning.

Since the reasoning member of this combination is the child, the intervention of a third person might be required to explain to each the differences in their personalities. This, however, could be done with good results if the mother were intelligent enough to realize the daughter's capabilities and permit her to exercise them. Such intelligent handling would establish mutual respect.

A third family problem which is not unusual may occur. Let us consider a family of five. The mother and two of the children, a boy and a girl, all had very similar endocrine patterns, whereas the father and third child had patterns which were like each other, but unlike those of the rest of the family.

Difficulty in this situation may arise due to the fact that the majority (mother and two children) had graphs that show an underactive thyroid, posterior pituitary and anterior pituitary, but all were andric. The father and third child had graphs with a slight underactivity of the posterior pituitary, marked overactivity of the anterior pituitary and gynic tendencies. The mother and two children were socially-minded, of average intelligence, ambitious and demanding. but because of their andricity they were dominating in manner. The father and one son were unusually intelligent, sympathetic and retiring in nature, more introvert than extrovert, but not at all socially-minded or ambitious in the material sense.

The only defense against the dominance and social-mindedness of the majority of this family which the father and one son could call upon, was to crawl further and further into their shells of self-sufficiency to withdraw rather than to force an issue. Consequently the father and son were looked upon as peculiar and in need of psychiatric help to make them like the rest of the family. However, they couldn't be made like the others; they came from a different cut-of-cloth, so to speak. Their needs were different, their outlook was different—different, but not wrong, not psychotic nor neurotic.

An intelligent handling of the situation would have been for the wife to praise the father's unusual earning capacity, to show his fine points to business associates while ignoring his social inadequacies (if they might be so-called). The wife's social-mindedness could have compensated for his lack in this regard, while his superior intelligence and finer sensibilities could have added greatly to their family life, to the culture and development of the children.

In marriage all too often the adding of one chemical to another is unsuccessful. If each has the power of four, so it remains. Marriages should mean an amalgamation of complementary powers, giving each the power of both—equal to eight. Occasionally one may even find two people who blend and complement each other so well that the two forces create a multiplication of power—equal to sixteen. That is the goal which understanding and appreciation of chemical differences, plus love, can achieve.

We are all born with a basic, potential personality, which is the result of our inherited endocrine pattern. Unfortunately, probably only about one person in a hundred has a perfect endocrine pattern. This leaves the majority of us with some degree of imbalance in the endocrine system. We are the product of several generations of poor diet which produces glandular deficiencies.

Since we are, in a sense, physically, emotionally, and mentally governed by our endocrine glands, it is important to consider what can be done to correct the situation for the sake of our marital partners and our children. First of all, proper diet will provide the raw materials to build normal functioning glands. This will automatically result in better health and bring about improvement in personality problems. If further correction is needed a scientific balancing of body chemistry by a specialist is recommended.

To attain the utmost in health is one step towards a successful marriage, but of equal importance is the mutual acceptance of the basic personality of our marriage partner. With this acceptance should come better understanding and a more conscious effort to fill each other's needs. Intuitively, we choose our mate with this in mind. Opposites do attract. Opposites can be blended into happy marriages.

However, these opposites in later years after the sexual attraction has lessened should both have their body chemistries corrected. Then they become alike in thinking, in disposition and are bound together by increased affection. They then become more as one. Their declining years may then become their happiest years.

IX. Cave-Man and Primitive Peoples
—What Lessons Do They Teach Us?

The misuse of civilization can be likened to a monster. It is consuming humans at an alarming rate; the toll is taken in cancer, arthritis, heart attacks, dental decay, and other diseases of the mouth, and what some term as stress and strain due to the fast pace of every day living. Probably the fast pace is just a convenient excuse. Man is perfectly geared and constructed to live at a fast pace provided he has a healthy body. Cave-man no doubt had to work hard to make a living, and probably had to work much harder than we do as he had no way of storing food for the future. He had to live from day to day with never more than a few days' food supply ahead. His greatest concern in life was getting enough food and keeping his family fed. He succeeded marvelously well as can be attested by the fact that we, his descendants, are here today.

Actually cave-man made possible the civilization which we have today because he took those first and most essential steps upon which a civilization could be built and expanded. Man is often defined as the tool making animal, and ancient cave-man made the first tools which were the precursor to all future technology. Now, in this discussion of civilization, it is to be stressed that civilization is a marvelous creation and development, but the misuse of civilization is a terrible thing in which the casualties can be counted in the millions in pain, suffering, and even death long before the natural life span has been reached. To understand how this has come about, it is best to first look at the mode of life of the savage—cave-man, our ancestors, and primitive peoples to see how they lived. From them we can learn much.

Little is known about the cave-man but there are enough of his remains to tell us that he lived a rugged, hardy life among all manner of dangers. We refer to these humans as Peking Man, Java Man, Neanderthal Man, and know that they lived from some half-million years ago or more, down until relatively recent times, perhaps down to 25,000 years ago or later. Cave-man made the first crude stone tools, lived in caves for protection from the elements and animals, and learned to use fire. During this period, called the Old Stone Age, the total population of humans must have been very small. Man's greatest danger was other animals that hunted him for food. In this period man was hunted as much as he hunted. He was food for many of the animals which were food for him. It was a dangerous and precarious life that he followed, yet, the skeletal remains which we have, show that he was very healthy. He had to be in order to survive.

Ancient cave-man was a flesh eating animal. Perhaps he ate a few wild fruits and plants which he found in the area, but for the most part he preferred meat. It was during this period that man learned to cook some of his food, though it would seem that he actually cooked very little of it. The current theory on how man developed a liking for cooked meat is interesting. It seems that in ancient times, just as sometimes happens today, lightning would start a forest fire. The burning forest trapped many animals, burning them to death, or if one prefers, cooking them.

It is logical to suppose that man ate the cooked animals as the food supply was short following a forest fire, and that he ate the cooked animals due to necessity. After repeating this a number of times, he began to like cooked flesh and having discovered how to make fire, one of the first great discoveries of our ancient ancestors, he then began to cook part of his food. However, when cave-man did cook his meat, it probably consisted of roasting it over an open fire.

He probably ate most of his meat raw, and that which

was cooked was most likely rare. We surmise that when game was not plentiful that cave-man then ate more of the available plant matter such as roots, nuts, berries, fruits, and greens. The variety of these plants and animals and frequency of their use depended on the geographical area.

We have ample evidence that cave-man lived primarily on meat. In his caves the bones of animals which he ate are numerous; they make up the so-called garbage of cave-man. Late in the Stone Age, man left us many beautiful cave paintings scattered over Central and Southern Europe and Africa. These paintings deal with the hunt and no doubt represent some type of divination to provide good hunting and plentiful game. At this stage of human existence, man depended almost entirely, if not completely, on meat for his subsistence. When the wild life and herds became scarce, he had to move on in search of them.

Thus man was in, what is termed by anthropologists, the hunting and gathering stage. In this period hunting was far more important than gathering. There were no domesticated animals, except possibly the dog, and it seems that the dog domesticated himself. The dog just took up with man and hung around his camp for scraps of meat and bones, whereas man found that the dog was useful to him in warning of approaching danger by barking and in hunting. Life in this period was not as savagely animal-like as one might imagine or as the cartoonist would have us believe. Man had to live by his wits alone to survive. For him life was hard in comparison with the way we live today. Cave-man did not look like an ape as he has often been pictured. Take a reconstruction of cave-man, give him a haircut and dress him in the present style of clothing and he hardly looks different from us at all. Man hasn't changed physiologically from ancient cave-man, and not at all from the men of 10,000 or more years ago. But, he has changed his mode of living. We smile and take comfort in feeling that we are so much better off than our ancestors, but are we? In some respects we have merely changed one set of dangers for another, though the ones we now have are primarily of our own creation. That is why we can do something about this situation if we make up our minds to do so. Man has the intelligence, but it remains to be seen if his application of this quality, which makes him human, will be applied. Had cave-man done otherwise we would not be here today. Are we doing the same for our descendants? This is the question that we need to ponder. The crucial theme of this book is the cause and prevention of degenerative diseases.

Man is basically a meat eater and meat alone, in most cases, can provide a very healthy diet for him. Dr. Vilhjalmur Stefansson, the most renowned authority on the Eskimo and his way of life, who spent years living with them reports that most Eskimos have dog teams and, since the people do not like the internal organs very well, that the dogs get most of them. Which ones they get depends on what animal is being eaten. For instance, if it is a caribou the dogs get the liver; if it is a seal the people eat the liver. In the case of the caribou the people first take the head, then the brisket, next the ribs and the pelvis meat. The dogs normally get everything from the inside of the body cavity except the kidneys and sometimes the heart; the dogs get the lungs, sweetbreads, stomach, intestines, but the Eskimos keep the fat from the intestines. They also give the dogs the hams, shoulders and the tenderloin, while they themselves eat the flesh off the ribs. It should be noted that the Eskimos eat lots of fat also.

Among many of the Eskimos, fish are also important and are eaten either raw or boiled. These Eskimos may be described as being in excellent health and with no manifestation of the degenerative diseases which constantly plague us, yet our dietitians considered their diet to be a very unhealthy one. They should have had scurvy, but it was not found nor did Dr. Stefansson in his years of living with the Eskimos on their diet contract scurvy. Actually fresh meat contains all the vitamin C that the body needs and this has been proven by later experiments. It must be borne in mind though, that although one can live very well on a meat diet, fat must go with it. If only lean meat is eaten, it will lead to sickness; lean meat and fat must be eaten together to give the proper balance that provides a complete diet. Even today, most people probably do not eat enough animal protein and certainly do not eat enough fat.

To prove the thesis that a complete meat diet is adequate for excellent health, Dr. Stefansson and Karsten Andersen submitted themselves to an experiment conducted by The Russell Sage Institute of Pathology at Bellevue Hospital and affiliated with the Medical College of Cornell University. For one year they ate nothing but meat in the ratio of 2 pounds of lean meat per day to ½ pound of fat. Dr. Stefansson, who had been on this diet for many years before beginning the experiments, was in excellent health both prior to and after the experiment. But, Karsten Anderson, who had been on an ordinary diet previously, was in a much better condition at the conclusion of the experiment than at the beginning. For those more interested in this aspect of nutrition, we highly recommend that you read Dr. Stefansson's book entitled *The Fat of the Land* published in 1956.

Now, that does not mean that everyone can live on meat alone, but most people can and would be in excellent health by doing so. However, many people do not have enough hydrochloric acid in their digestive system, and they do not handle meat too well. The point is that ancient cave-man lived almost entirely on meat and was in excellent health. A contemporary race, the Eskimo, also lives on, or did until recently, an almost complete meat diet. He was surprisingly healthy with practically none of the degenerative diseases which plague us. Some authorities gave the explanation as being hereditary or racial. They stated that the reason the Eskimo was so healthy was due as much to his race as to his diet. Yet, the results of the experiment conducted with Dr. Stefansson and Mr. Anderson and also their years of living with the Eskimo on his native diet, dispelled such an explanation. The reason lies primarily in diet. Today, in the areas where the Eskimo has gone on a civilized diet—the sugar, refined grains, white flour, milk and coffee—he has begun to suffer from rampant degenerative disease. He had a good heredity which is important, but a faulty and destructive diet can, and does bring about degeneration rapidly. Also, susceptibility to infectious diseases has been increased, and the Eskimo today is a disappearing race.

The Eskimos live in the Stone Age, and from them we can surmise a great deal about the mode of living of ancient cave-man. Of all the adaptations made by man to his environment, the Eskimos have made one of the most successful. Up until very recently in this century, if people from other parts of the world wanted to live in the Arctic, they had to adapt to the way and life of the Eskimo in order to survive. Dr. Stefansson and Mr. Anderson, as have numerous others, discovered this, and what is most surprising, after living on the Eskimo diet, they found that they were healthier than they were before. We have a lot to learn from the primitive peoples of the world of which the Eskimos are only one group.

The Old Stone Age did not provide man with a completely wonderful life. For one thing, although he had a good diet when he could find food, there were no doubt times when food was very scarce and starvation was always just around the corner. Cave-man had to spend so much time in search of food that he had little time for anything else. He faced constant danger too from predatory animals.

To use the phrase of the late 19th century philosopher, Herbert Spencer, this period for man was one of "survival of the fittest." The Old Stone Age lasted a very long time, perhaps a million years, but it was during this period that man made the initial discoveries that made civilization and a larger population possible. During the Old Stone Age the human population was no doubt very small, and it had to be by necessity due to the mode of living. The food supply was limited and man had to wander from place to place to follow the game he hunted. Once man learned how to have a more stable and dependable food supply civilization began to develop rapidly.

This period of development passed through several stages and it was not uniform the world over. Today, there are still primitive people living in the Stone Age; for example the Australian aborigines, the Eskimos, Indians of the Amazon Basin, and some groups in Africa and Asia. One of the biggest problems of the world today is with the so-called undeveloped countries which comprise those nations that have not become industrialized. Industrialization can either be a blessing to these nations or it can bring the same problems that we face, namely a population becoming more and more plagued by degenerative diseases primarily due to faulty nutrition and poor heredity caused by a bad diet over several generations.

From the Old Stone Age man passed into what is termed the New Stone Age. Man learned to grow some of his own food and to raise some animals, thus gaining a measure of control over his food supply. He could even produce a surplus which would free some people to devote themselves exclusively to other occupations such as making pottery, weapons, weaving cloth, etc. Civilization had begun.

This period did not begin immediately with agriculture and animal husbandry, but it developed gradually and in different ways over the world. The first stage in which man began to grow his food is termed gardening or horticulture which means specifically that man did not use draft animals in the growing of food. All gardening peoples had some domesticated animals for food, but they were not used in plowing and preparing land for cultivation.

Gardening began in the New Stone Age and some very high civilizations evolved with this method of growing food. One very good example is the Inca Empire of South America where one of the greatest civilizations known was carried to its height of development. It is from the Incas that we get some of our common and basic foods of today such as the potato, lima beans, corn, sweet potato and peanuts. The Incas had huge herds of domesticated llamas and alpacas, great flocks of muscovy ducks and each household also had guinea pigs for food. Probably the main reason that the Incas did not use draft animals in their horticulture is because none were present. Yet, at the time of the conquest, their gardening type of agriculture was much superior to the true agriculture of Europe. And, the land was more productive during this period than it was under the Spaniards who conquered the Inca Empire in 1533. From that time on the Indian population began to suffer, but it may also be noted that the native population which has remained to this day on the native diet is much healthier than those who have adopted the European diet.

At the same time that gardening or agriculture began, another form of economy which provided a food surplus and insured stability of food, pastorialism, was introduced. Now, as has been pointed out previously, all gardening or agriculture peoples had some domesticated animals, but their major basic food supply came from the earth. Actually, all of man's food supply is based on vegetable matter. He either eats foods that belong to the plant family or he eats animals which are grown and fattened on vegetable matter, such as cattle. Man must have animal protein to be robust and healthy; he cannot subsist in a healthy state on plant foods alone. A good example of this is the Hindu population of southern India. The biological structure of their diet is seriously undermined by their extreme shortage of high-value protein, since their religion prohibits the eating of meat. This deficiency has set in motion a series of ill effects which has lead to a severe degradation of the race.

In contrast the Sihks, who live in Pemjab in Northern India, are tall, have more robust physiques, appear more vigorous and have good health. Their diet consists of whole wheat bread and animal protein in contrast to the rice and vegetable menu of the south. The almost complete absence of animal proteins in the Hindu's diet accounts for his short stature, his low energy and his great susceptibility to disease.

It is apparent that agriculture made civilization possible, and as long as man eats a good diet consisting of wholesome plant products and animal protein in the proper proportions, he will have the natural diet which is necessary for good health.

In order for a civilization to exist and perpetuate itself,

it is necessary for that civilization to have a technology for securing sufficient food to satisfy the wants of its people. Agriculture and the domestication of animals made that possible. Note though that the word "wants" rather than "needs" is used because customs tend to create wants for particular kinds of edible substances and to suppress, minimize or prohibit others. A civilization must provide sufficient food to maintain a degree of health and vigor in its people, but customs often prevent a people from using the resources available to it. A good example of this is India where the Hindu religion, was previously cited. But it is not necessary to go to India for an example. The United States will suffice, where people prefer to eat refined sugar and bleached flour which has been robbed of all vitamins, minerals and enzymes rather than those foods necessary to health. In many civilizations the staple diet may be largely determined by the natural resources of the environment and the available technology, but in nearly all civilizations people make efforts to secure some foods out of all proportion to their nutritive value and often reject or even forbid the eating of foods highly prized by other civilizations. Again sugar can be cited in our civilization, a food which is actually harmful yet highly prized and constitutes such a basic part of the American diet that people will go to almost any means to get it; coffee is another. Just remember the days of rationing in World War II when sugar and coffee were rationed with the result that hoarding, took place and there were even black market dealings in these products. Another example is that of shrimp. We relish shrimp but reject grasshoppers which are highly prized as a delicacy by the aboriginal Australians. We eat what we do primarily because of custom.

Man is distinguished from other animals chiefly by his intelligence which has endowed him with mechanical abilities. One major part of civilization is only a finer degree of applied mechanical ability. This in itself is merely the application or use by the multitudes of what was discovered by the few. Strip us of our clothes, our houses, our automobiles, our knives and forks and we would hardly be any different from cave-man whom we think of as living in the most abject and depraved conditions. Yet, as pointed out previously, it was cave-man who made civilization possible. Perhaps language was rudimentary. Of all the animals, man is the only one who has language—or languages to be more exact—the ability to symbolize making communication possible. Inventions are worthless if one cannot teach others of the invention. This is, in short, communication. Civilization is the combined experiences of others taught to the individual and passed on from generation to generation. Knowledge is cumulative and as such man can accept that of the past, utilize it in the present and built upon it for future needs.

Every discovery or invention made has been based upon numerous discoveries and inventions made by past generations. A large portion of civilization falls within the field of mechanics in which our progress has been astounding. Of man's million or more years on earth, practically all of the great mechanical discoveries have been made within the last five to ten thousand years, and the latter figure is not a conservative one. Yet, apparently to judge from man's fossil remains and from what we learn from the archaeologists and history, man's intelligence has not increased at all. Perhaps this is not important as man does not use much of the intelligence with which he has been endowed. Of the great and powerful civilizations of the past, practically everyone of them fell not due to outside pressure and conquest, but due to internal deterioration and disintegration. Often they were conquered, but the conqueror merely dealt the death blow to an already decadent and dying civilization. A good example of this was the Inca Empire of South America. When the Spaniards arrived it was engaged in a civil war which had weakened the whole structure of the state. India could never have been subdued by the British had she been a unified country rather than one made up of hundreds of warring little kingdoms and principalities. Of all the great nations of the ancient world, only one remains—China, who had her beginning in 1750 B.C. and has had a continuing civilization ever since. Egypt, Assyria, Babylonia, Greece, Rome and all the others ceased to exist long ago. Each left us a legacy and our civilization is more materially comfortable because of the contributions of these past civilizatons, yet perhaps the greatest lesson we could learn from them would be the facts pertaining to the causes of their decline and fall. In every case the downfall was caused by the civilization itself.

In the period from September 1948 to November 1958, 40 percent of all the young men drafted for service in our armed forces were rejected for physical, mental or moral reasons. It is alarming to report that the rate is increasing; it reached 48.8 per cent in 1959. The young men of the U.S. are the cream of the crop, the progenitors of the future and the ones who must build that better world of tomorrow that we so hope for and dream about. At the present, over 48 per cent of them are unfit for military service. The facts do not look so bright for the future. It is time that we asked ourselves why so many young men are not physically and mentally sound, particularly when the unhealthy constitute over two-fifths of the draft age population of the U.S. The trend can be reversed if only we will use our scientific knowledge wisely for the benefit of mankind and stop our flagrant abuse of technology which has changed us from a "have-not" country to a "have" nation, so that today we are the richest nation that the world has ever known. But, we are very vulnerable, just like all the rich and pompous empires and nations of the past, to creeping corrosion, luxury, and the unwise use of our technology. Sedentarianism, indooritis, and push buttonism are rendering us weak. It is getting so that the average American is forgetting that he has legs with which to walk; if he needs to walk over a block, and a very short one at that, he decides that he must ride. We are told that the present generation is the tallest, heaviest and most diseasefree in all of our history, but the truth of the matter is that our youth are being subtly victimized by an age of standardization, mechanization, urbanization and complete materialism. Even though infectious diseases are very well controlled, the degenerative diseases to come are apparent when over 48 per cent of our young men are not fit for military service of any kind.

Degenerative disease is on the increase. The ony measurement we have had of the progress of degenerative diseases are the statistics tabulated by insurance companies showing the yearly increase which is constantly mounting. These are not entirely convincing for it can be pointed out that more people are living to the age of susceptibility to diseases than formerly, because of the great strides made by medical science in combating infectious diseases. Control of infectious diseases and infant mortality, has statistically lengthened the span that an individual may expect to live. Often people get the wrong impression of this because they fail to realize how important is the overall figure when infant mortality is cut to a very small percentage per thousand. In olden times, if a person got through infancy and childhood, he ran a pretty good chance of living to a ripe old age. So, we cannot state that more people are dying of heart diseases, and the other degenerative diseases just because they are living longer; that is only one part of the story and too many are dying in the prime of life—in their forties and fifties. These premature deaths can be averted if only we will utilize our scientific knowledge wisely and take care of our bodies accordingly.

We think of ourselves as individuals but we are also links in a long chain; a chain that goes back to the beginning of man. If over a period of a hundred years each link in the chain became one per cent weaker than its predecessor, the end of the race would be near. And yet, one per cent weakening in each generation would be so slight as to be imperceptible. What is actually happening is that the increase in disability is so rapid that it can be seen. Grandchildren in general have less body resistance and are more subject to ills than their grandparents were at a like age. If we do not wish to become a subjugated people or extinct, we must go back to the rules of nutrition—no harmful things and all of the essentials.

Our bodies are today the same mechanical contrivances that they were thousands of years ago, and thousands of generations ago the chain was very strong. We talk about our heredity—we brag about it—but what we have was given to us—what we should be sure of is that we pass along to the next generation as good as we have received.

In this time of world upheaval with one war barely over, everyone fearing the next and minor skirmishes being reported daily, it well behooves those who bear the burden of perpetuating the race to see that the stock is strengthened by all the means within their reach. The future of civilization is dependent not only upon the survival of democracy, but upon the propagation of nations of peoples healthy in body and mind, and at peace with each other because of mutual understanding and respect.

Bibliography

Abrahamson, E. M., and Pezet, A. W. *Body, Mind and Sugar,* Henry Holt and Co., New York, 1951.

Albrecht, Wm. A.; Gay, Lee Pettit; Jones, G. S., "Trace Elements, Allergies and Soil Deficiencies," *The Journal of Applied Nutrition,* Vol. 13, No. 1, 1960.

——: *Soil Fertility and Animal Health,* Fred Hahne Printing Co., Webster City, Iowa, 1958.

——: *Protein Deficiencies via Soil Deficiencies,* Department of Soils, College of Agriculture, University of Missouri, 1951.

Alexander, F. Mathias, *The Universal Constant in Living,* New York, E. P. Dutton & Co., Inc., 1942.

Ashley-Montagu, F. M. *Man, His First Million Years,* The World Publishing Co., Cleveland, Ohio, 1957.

——: *An Introduction to Physical Anthropology,* Charles C. Thomas Pub., Springfield, 1960.

Balfour, E. D., *The Living Soil,* Devin-Adair Co., New York, 1950.

Beach, Frank A., *Hormones and Behavior,* Paul B. Hoeber, Inc., New York, 1948.

Beals, Ralph and Hoijer, Harry, *An Introduction to Anthropology,* The Macmillan Co., New York, 1953.

Benedict, F. G. and Steggerda, Morris, *The Food of the Present Day Maya Indians of Yucatan,* Pub. 546, Contrib. 18, Carnegie Institute, Washington.

Bicknell, Franklin, and Prescott, Frederick, *The American and His Food,* University of Chicago Press, Chicago, 1941.

Biskind, Morton S., "The Technic of Nutritional Therapy," *The Journal of Applied Nutrition,* Vol. 13, No. 1, 1960.

Bodansky, M. and Bodansky O., *Biochemistry of Disease,* Second Edition, The Macmillan Co., New York, 1952.

Boyd, William C., *Genetics and The Races of Man*, Boston University Press, 1950.

Broderick, F. W., *The Principles of Dental Medicine*, The C. V. Mosby Co., St. Louis, 1936.

———: *The Principles of Dental Medicine*, C. V. Mosby Co., St. Louis, 1939.

Burket, Lester W., *Oral Medicine*, J. B. Lippincott Co., Philadelphia, 1946.

Calder, Ritchie, *Medicine and Man*, The New American Library, New York, 1958.

Carrel, Alexis, *Man, the Unknown*, Harper, New York, 1935.

Castro, Josue de, *The Geography of Hunger*, Little, Brown & Co., Boston, 1952.

Cheraskin, E.; Flynn, F. H. and Fess, L. R., "Blood Sugar Levels During the Dental Experience I, Blood Sugar Level in the Waiting Room," *Journal of Oral Surgery, Anesthesia and Hospital Dental Service*, Vol. 18, January, 1960.

———, Brunson, C.: "The Relationship of Fasting Blood Glucose to Oral Symptoms," *The Journal of Applied Nutrition*, Vol. 13, No. 1, 1960.

———, Flynn, F. H.; Hutto, A. C.; Fless, L. R.; Huffstutler, B. B. and Brocker, C. E., "The Alabama Study of Maternal Ascorbic Acid Nutrition," *Alabama Dental Review*, Spring Issue, 1960.

———, Brunson, C.; Sheridan, Jr., R. C.; Flynn, F. H.; Hutto A. C.; Keller, S. M. and Basile, J.: "The Normal Glucose Tolerance Pattern: The Development of Blood Glucose Normality by an Analysis of Oral Symptoms," *The Journal of Periodontology*, Vol. 31, April, 1960.

Childe, V. Gordon, *Man Makes Himself*, The Rationalist Press Association, London, 1936.

Climate and Man, Yearbook of Agriculture, 1941, U. S. Government Printing Office, 1941.

Comas, Juan, *Manual of Physical Anthropology*, Charles C. Thomas Pub., Springfield, 1960.

Davidson, Sir. Stanley; Meiklejohn A. P. and Passmore R., *Human Nutrition and Dietetics*, The Williams and Wilkins Co., Baltimore, 1959.

Davis, A. Edward, *Cataract, Its Preventive and Medical Treatment*, F. A. Davis Co., Philadelphia, 1938.

Dolger, H., from Soffer, L.: *Diseases of the Endocrine Glands,* Lea & Febiger, Philadelphia, 1951.

Downing, John Godwin, *The Cutaneous Manifestations of Systemic Diseases,* Charles C. Thomas, Pub., Springfield, 1954.

Draper, George; Dupertuis, C. W., and Caughey, J. L., Jr., *Human Constitution in Clinical Medicine,* Harper and Bros., New York, 1944.

Drummond, Jack Cecil, and Willoraham, Anne, *The Englishman's Food: A History of Five Centuries of English Diet,* Jonathan Cape. Ltd., 1939.

Dunn, L. C. and Dobzhansky, L. C., *Heredity, Race and Society,* The New American Library of World Literature, Inc., New York, 1946.

Edsall, John T., editor, *Enzymes and Enzyme Systems, Their State in Nature,* Harvard University Press, Cambridge, 1951.

Engel, R. W. and Copeland, D. H., *Cancer Research,* Vol. 12, University of Chicago Press, 1952.

Female Sex Hormone Therapy, Medical Research Division, The Schering Corporation, 1941.

Food, Yearbook of Agriculture, 1939, U. S. Government Printing Office, 1939.

Food and Life, Yearbook of Agriculture, 1939, U. S. Government Printing Office, 1939.

Fried, Morton H., *Readings in Anthropology,* Vol. I & II, Thomas Y. Corwell Co., New York, 1959.

Gann, T. W. F., *The Maya Indians of Southern Yucatan and Northern British Honduras,* Bureau of American Ethnology, Bull. No. 64, Washington, 1918.

Garn, Stanley M., *Readings on Race,* Charles C. Thomas, Pub., Springfield, 1959.

Glandular Physiology and Therapy, Council on Pharmacy and Chemistry of the American Medical Association, Fifth Edition, J. B. Lippincott Co., Philadelphia, 1954.

Goldschmidt, Walter, *Man's Way,* Henry Holt & Co., Inc., New York, 1959.

Goldzieher, Max A., *The Adrenal Glands in Health and Disease,* F. A. Davis Co., Philadelphia, 1944.

Gordon, Gilbert S. and Lisser, H., *Endocrinology in Clinical Practice,* The Year Book Publishers, Inc., Chicago, 1953.

Gordon, Edgar S., and Sevringhaus, Elmer L., *Vitamin Therapy in General Practice*. The Year Book Publishers, Inc., Chicago, 1942.

Green, David E., *Currents in Biochemical Research*, Interscience Publishers, New York, 1956.

Grollman, Arthur, *Essentials of Endocrinology*, J. B. Lippincott Co., Philadelphia, 1947.

Hamblen, E. C., *Endocrine Gynecology*, Charles C. Thomas, Baltimore, 1939.

Handbook of Nutrition, A Symposium Prepared Under the Auspices of the Council on Foods and Nutrition of the American Medical Association, 1943.

Harrow, Benjamin, *Biochemistry*, W. B. Saunders and Co., Philadelphia, 1938.

Harrower, Henry R., *An Endocrine Handbook*, The Harrower Laboratory, Inc., Glendale, California, 1939.

Haurowitz, Belix, *Chemistry and Biology of Proteins*, Academic Press, Inc., New York, 1950.

Hawkins, Harold F., *Applied Nutrition*, Institute Press, Gardena, California, 1940.

Herskovits, Melville J., *Man and His Works*, Alfred A. Knopf, New York, 1951.

Heyningen, W. E. van., *Bacterial Toxins*, Charles C. Thomas, Springfield, Illinois, 1959.

Hoebel, E. Adamson, *Man in the Primitive World*, McGraw-Hill Book Co., New York, 1958.

——, Jennings, Jesse D. and Smith, Elmer R., *Readings in Anthropology*, McGraw-Hill Book Co., Inc., New York, 1955.

Hoffman, Jacob, *Female Endocrinology including sections of the Male*, W. B. Saunders Co., Philadelphia, 1944.

Hooten, Ernest Albert, *Up From The Ape*, The Macmillan Co., New York, 1946.

——: *Apes, Man and Morons*, Putnam, New York, 1937.

Howard, Sir Albert, *The Soil and Health, Farming and Gardening for Health or Disease*, Devin-Adair Co., New York, 1947.

——: *An Agricultural Testament*, Oxford University Press, New York, 1940.

Huntington, Ellsworth, *Principles of Human Geography*, John Wiley & Sons, New York, 1947.

———: *Mainsprings of Civilization*, John Wiley & Sons, New York, 1945.

Huxley, Julian, *Evolution in Action*, Harper & Bros., New York, 1953.

———: *Evolution: The Modern Synthesis*, Harper & Bros., New York, 1953.

Kahn, Fritz, *Man in Structure and Function*, Vol. I & II, Alferd A. Knopf, New York, 1953.

Klein, H. and Palmer, C. E., *Dental Caries In American Indian Children*, U. S. Public Health Bulletin No. 239, Washington, 1937.

Korn, Noel and Smith, Harry Reece, Edited by, *Human Evolution*, Henry Holt & Co., New York, 1959.

Kroeber, A. L., Editor, *Anthropology Today*, University of Chicago Press, 1953.

Lee, Royal, "Civilization and Cancer," *Natural Food and Farming*, Vol. 7, No. 2, Atlanta, Texas, July, 1960.

Leicester, Henry M., *Biochemistry of the Teeth*, C. V. Mosby Co., St. Louis, 1949.

Lieb, Clarence W., "The Effects of an Exclusive Long-Continued Meat Diet, Based on the History, Experience and Clinical Survey of Vilhjalmur Stefansson, Arctic Explorer," *Journal of the American Medical Association*, July 3, 1926.

———: "The Effects on Human Beings on a Twelve Month Exclusive Meat Diet," *Journal of the American Medical Association*, July 6, 1929.

———: "A Year's Exclusive Meat Diet and Seven Years Later," *American Journal of Digestive Diseases and Nutrition*, Vol. II, No. 8.

———, Stefansson, V. and Thomas, Wm. A., "Meat Diet in Health and Disease," *American Medical Association reprint*, 1927.

Longgood, William, *The Poisons in Your Food*, Simon & Schuster, New York, 1960.

Mack, Pauline Berry, *Nutrition of Older Girls and Boys*, Texas State College for Women, Denton, Texas, 1955.

Mackarness, Richard, *Eat Fat and Grow Slim*, Doubleday & Co., Inc., New York, 1959.

Malcom, John Erskin, *Blood Pressure Sounds and Their Meanings*, Charles C. Thomas, London, 1957.

Male Sex Hormone Therapy, First Edition, Medical Research Division, The Scherine Corp., 1941.

Marriott, H. L., *Water and Salt Depletion,* Charles C. Thomas Pub., Springfield, Ill., 1950.

McCarrison, Sir Robert and Sinclair, H. M., *Nutrition and Health,* Faber and Faber, London, 1953.

McCarrison, Robert, *Studies in Deficiency Disease,* Oxford Medical Publications, Henry Frowde and Hodder & Stoughton, London, 1945.

McClellan, Walter S., "The Effect of the Prolonged Use of Exclusive Meat Diets on Two Men," *Journal of the American Dietetic Association,* December, 1930.

McCollum, E. V. and J. Ernestine Becker, *Food, Nutrition and Health,* Third Edition, Baltimore, 1934.

Medical Research: *A Midcentury Survey,* Vol. 1 & 2, The American Foundation, Little, Brown & Co., Boston, 1955.

Metabolic Individuality and Diagnosis of Degenerative Disease, Lakeside Laboratories, Inc., Milwaukee, 1951.

Miller, Fred D., *Open Door to Health,* The Devin-Adair Co., New York, 1959.

Miller, Heymen R. and Fulton, John F., *Central Autonomic Regulations in Health and Disease,* Grune & Stratton, New York, 1942.

Missenard, Andre, *In Search of Man,* Hawthorn Books, Inc., New York, 1957.

Monier—Williams, G. W., *Trace Elements in Food,* John Wiley & Sons, Inc., New York, 1949.

Morley, Sylvanus G., *The Ancient Maya,* Stanford University Press, Stanford, 1946.

Moschcowitz, Eli., *Biology of Disease,* Grune & Stratton, New York, 1948.

Murdock, George Peter, *Our Primitive Contemporaries,* The Macmillan Co., New York, 1934.

Norman, N. Philip, "The Triad Disease," *Mankind's No. 1 Killer,* Lee Foundation for Nutritional Research, Milwaukee, 1958.

Ochsner, Alton, *Smoking and Health,* Julian Messner, Inc., New York, 1954.

Osborne, Fairfield, *Our Plundered Planet,* Little, Brown & Co., Boston, 1948.

Ott, John, *My Ivory Cellar, The Story of Time-Lapse Photography*, Twentieth Century Press, Inc., Chicago, 1958.

Packard, Vance, *The Hidden Persuaders*, Pocket Books, Inc., New York, 1957.

Page, Melvin E., "Conservation of Edentulous Alveolar Process," *The Journal of the American Dental Association*, March, 1936.

——: "Necessity for Endocrine Treatment in Successful Prosthesis," *The Journal of the American Dental Association*, March, 1936.

——: "Practical Application of Preventive Dental Medicine," *Nutrition and Dental Health*, January, February, and March, 1938.

——: "Dental Caries," *American Dental Association*, 1941.

——: "Dentistry from the Inside," *Dental Items of Interest*, April, 1944.

——: "Glands and Dentistry," *Dental Items of Interest*, April, 1944.

——: "Sugar Metabolism," *Dental Items of Interest*, July, 1944.

——: *Young Minds with Old Bodies*, Bruce Humphries, Inc., Boston, 1944.

——; *Degeneration—Regeneration*, Page Foundation, Inc., 1949.

——, Brooks, D. L., and Daly, R. B., "Body Chemistry in Health and Disease," *Dental Digest*, September, 1953 through June, 1954, Reprinted in monograph form by Page Foundation, Inc., 1954.

Pappenheimer, Alwin M., *Vitamin E Deficiency*, Charles C. Thomas Pub., Springfield, 1948.

Paschkis, Karl E.; Rakoff, Abraham E.; Cantarow, Abraham, *Clinical Endocrinology*, Paul E. Hoeber, Inc., New York, 1954.

Peterson, Frederick, *Ancient Mexico*, G. P. Putnam's Sons, New York, 1959.

Picton, Lionel, *Nutrition and the Soil: Thoughts on Feeding*, Devin-Adair Co., New York, 1949.

"Preliminary Report of the Committee on Interstate and Foreign Commerce," *House Report No. 1338*, March 16, 1954.

Price, Weston A., *Nutrition and Physical Degeneration,* The American Academy of Applied Nutrition, Los Angeles, 1939.

Pruden, Bonnie, *Is Your Child Really Fit?* Harper Bros., New York, 1956.

Quigley, D. T., *The National Malnutrition,* The Lee Foundation for Nutritional Research, Milwaukee, 1943.

Ragan, Charles and Snyder, Arthur I., *Rheumatoid Arthritis,* The Year Book Publishers, Chicago, 1955.

Rawson, Rulon W., *Hyperthyroidism,* The Year Book Pub., Chicago, 1955.

Roberts, Sam E., *Ear, Nose and Throat Dysfunctions due to Deficiencies and Imbalances,* Charles C. Thomas, Springfield, 1957.

Rodale, J. I., *Organic Gardening,* Hanover House, Garden City, New York, 1959.

——: *The Healthy Hunzas,* Rodale Press, Emmaus, Pa., 1949.

Rorty, James, Editor, *American Fluoridation Experiment,* Devin-Adair Co., New York, 1957.

Rubel, Louis L., *The GP and the Endocrine Glands,* Decator, Ill., 1959.

Samuels, Jules, *Endogenous Endocrinotherapy,* 11th Edition, N. V. Cycloscoop, Publisher, Amsterdam, 1960.

Schoenheimer, Rudolph, *The Dynamic State of the Body Constituents,* Harvard University Press, Cambridge, Mass., 1942.

Sears, Victor H., *New Teeth for Old,* University of Utah Press, 1950.

Service, Elman R., *A Profile of Primitive Culture,* Harper Bros., New York, 1958.

Seyle, Hans, *The Physiology and Pathology of Exposure to Stress,* ACTA, Inc., Medical Publishers, Montreal, 1950.

Shaw, J. C. M., "Dental Caries in Native Children," *Journal American Dental Association,* 19:2219, 1932.

Sheldon, William H., *Atlas of Men,* Harper & Bros., New York, 1954.

——: Stevens, S. S., Tucker, W. B., *The Varieties of Human Physique,* Harper & Bros., New York, 1940.

Sherman, Henry C., *Food and Health,* Macmillan & Co., New York, 1941.

Shohl, Alfred T., *Mineral Metabolism,* Reinhold Publishing Co., New York, 1939.

Simpson, George Gaylor, *The Meaning of Evolution,* Yale University Press, 1949.

Soil, Yearbook of Agriculture, 1957, U. S. Government Printing Office, 1957.

Soils and Men, Yearbook of Agriculture, 1938, U. S. Government Printing Office, 1938.

Stefansson, Vilhjalmur, *The Fat of the Land,* The Macmillan Co., New York, 1957.

———: "Food of the Ancient and Modern Stone Age Man," *Journal of the American Dietetic Association,* Vol. 13, No. 2, July, 1937.

———: *My Life with the Eskimo,* The Macmillan Co., New York, 1951.

Steggerda, Morris, *Maya Indians of Yucatan,* Publication 531, Carnegie Institute, Washington, 1941.

Stephen, Robert M., "Relative Importance of Polysaccharides, Disaccharides, and Monosaccharides in the Production of Caries," *Journal of American Dental Association,* Vol. 37, November, 1948.

Stern, Frances, *Applied Dietetics,* The Williams & Wilkins Co., Baltimore, 1943.

Storer, John H., *The Web of Life,* Devin-Adair Co., New York, 1953.

Survey of Food and Nutrition Research in the United States of America 1952-53. Prepared by Food and Nutrition Board, National Research Council, U. S. Government Printing Office, Washington, 1954.

Sutton, Philip R. N., *Fluoridation,* Cambridge University Press, New York, 1959.

Tax, Sol: Eiseley, C. Loren; Rouse, Irving, and Voegelin, Carl F., *An Appraisal of Anthropology Today,* University of Chicago Press, 1953.

Thoma, K. H., "Oral Manifestations of Disease," *Journal American Dental Association,* Vol. 29, No. 2, 1942.

Thompson, J. Eric S., *The Rise and Fall of Maya Civilization,* University of Oklahoma Press, Norman, 1954.

Tolstoi, Edward, "The Effect of an Exclusive Meat Diet on the Chemical Constituents of the Blood," *Journal of Biological Chemistry,* September, 1929.

Toynbee, Arnold J., *Civilization on Trial*, Oxford University Press, New York, 1948.
——: *A Study of History*, Abridgment of Volumes I-VI by D. C. Somervell, Oxford University Press, New York, 1946.

Ucko, H., *Endocrines Diagnosis*, Staples Press, London, 1951.

Van Hook, Andres, *Sugar, It's Production, Technology, and Uses*, Ronald Press Co., New York, 1949.
——: *Sugar*, The Rodale Press, New York, 1949.

Wickenden, Leonard, *Our Daily Poison*, The Devin-Adair Co., New York, 1955.
Wiley, Harvey W., *History of a Crime Against the Food Law*, the author, Washington, 1929.
Wilkins, Robert W. *Essential Hypertension*, The Year Book Publishers, Chicago, 1955.
Williams, Roger, *Alcoholism: The Nutritional Approach*, University of Texas Press, 1959.
——: *Biochemical Individuality*, John Wiley & Sons, Inc., New York, 1956.
——: *Free and Unequal*, University of Texas Press, Austin, 1953.
Wintrobe, Maxwell, M., *The Anemias*, The Year Book Pub., Chicago, 1955.
Wood, H. Curtis, Jr., *Overfed but Undernourished,* Exposition Press, Inc., New York, 1959.
Wrench, G. T., *The Wheel of Health*, The C. W. Daniel Co., Ltd., London, 1938.

Yanovsky, E., *Food Plants of the North American Indians*, U. S. Department of Agriculture, Misc. Pub., No. 237, Washington, 1936.

HEALTH POWER IS YOURS
WITH THESE NEW BOOKS!

☐ **SINUSITIS, BRONCHITIS AND EMPHYSEMA**
  (Clifford Quick)   **$1.95**

☐ **YOUR BODY IS YOUR BEST DOCTOR**
  (Melvin E. Page, D.D.S.)   **$1.25**

☐ **GO AHEAD AND LIVE** (Mildred Loomis)   **95ᶜ**

☐ **KNOW YOUR NUTRITION** (Linda Clark)   **$3.50**

☐ **RECIPE FOR SURVIVAL** (Doris Grant)   **$3.95**

☐ **YOUR KEYS TO RADIANT HEALTH**
  (William E. Dankenbring)   **$1.95**

☐ **THE HEALING NEEDLES** (Charles Ewart)   **$1.25**

☐ **HEALING BENEFITS OF ACUPRESSURE**
  (F.M. Houston, D.C.)   **$4.95**

☐ **YOUR NATURAL HEALTH SAMPLER**
  (Linda Clark and others)   **$1.25**

☐ **YOUR WATER AND YOUR HEALTH**
  (Allen E. Banik and Carlson Wade)   **$1.25**

☐ **EAT THE WEEDS** (Ben Charles Harris)   **$1.25**

☐ **DIET HEALTH CARD** (T.L. Cleave, M.D.)   **$1.00**

Buy them at your local health or book store or use this coupon.

- -

Keats Publishing, Inc. (P.O. Box 876), New Canaan, Conn. 06840   75-E
Please send me the books I have checked above. I am enclosing
$____ (add 35ᶜ to cover postage and handling). Send check or
money order—no cash or C.O.D.'s please.

Mr/Mrs/Miss_____

Address _____

City _____ State _____ Zip_____
(Allow three weeks for delivery)

COOKBOOKS ON NATURAL HEALTH
. . . To Help You Eat Better for Less!

☐ **ADD A FEW SPROUTS** (Martha H. Oliver) — **$1.50**

☐ **WHOLE GRAIN BAKING SAMPLER**
   (Beatrice Trum Hunter) — **$2.25**

☐ **MRS. APPLEYARD'S KITCHEN** (L.A. Kent) — **$3.50**

☐ **MRS. APPLEYARD'S SUMMER KITCHEN**
   (L.A. Kent & E.K. Gay) — **$3.50**

☐ **MRS. APPLEYARD'S WINTER KITCHEN**
   (L.A. Kent & E.K. Gay) — **$3.50**

☐ **BETTER FOODS FOR BETTER BABIES** (Gena Larson) — **95ᶜ**

☐ **GOOD FOODS THAT GO TOGETHER** (Elinor L. Smith) — **$2.95**

☐ **MEALS AND MENUS FOR ALL SEASONS** (Agnes Toms) — **$1.25**

☐ **NATURAL FOODS BLENDER COOKBOOK**
   (Frieda Nusz) — **$1.25**

☐ **GOLDEN HARVEST PRIZE WINNING RECIPES**
   (ed. by B.T. Hunter) — **$1.25**

☐ **SOYBEANS FOR HEALTH** (Philip Chen) — **$1.25**

☐ **FOOD AND FELLOWSHIP** (Elizabeth S. Pistole) — **95ᶜ**

☐ **MENNONITE COMMUNITY COOKBOOK**
   (Mary Emma Showalter) — **$1.25**

☐ **EAT THE WEEDS** (Ben Charles Harris) — **$1.25**

Buy them at your local health or book store or use this coupon.

Keats Publishing, Inc. (P.O. Box 876), New Canaan, Conn. 06840 75-G
Please send me the books I have checked above. I am enclosing
$____ (add 35ᶜ to cover postage and handling). Send check or
money order—no cash or C.O.D.'s please.
Mr/Mrs/Miss_____

Address _____

City _____ State _____ Zip_____
                    (Allow three weeks for delivery)   Printed in U.S.A.